The Burning Mouth Syndrome

The Burning Mouth Syndrome

Isaäc van der Waal
Professor,
Department of Oral and Maxillofacial Surgery
and Oral Pathology,
Free University / ACTA,
Amsterdam, The Netherlands

Munksgaard

Cover and composition by Jens Lund Kirkegaard
Printed in Denmark by P.J.Schmidt A/S, Vojens
ISBN 87-16-10381-5

Preface

The Burning Mouth Syndrome (BMS) is an enigmatous condition for both the patient and the clinician.

When the syndrome is not recognized as such, the patient may become exposed to a variety of treatment modalities, including dental and surgical procedures, which are not beneficial and often even aggravate the problem.

The possible etiologic role of psychogenic causes of the burning sensation is widely discussed in the literature, but has not led to solid evidence of such a cause-and-effect relationship. Therefore, the patient with symptoms of BMS should be protected from being, often needlessly and incorrectly, referred for psychiatric treatment.

Management of patients suffering from BMS requires patience and understanding from the doctor's side. By following a step by step approach, as outlined in the book, a number of patients will be treated successfully, while in others an apparently unbearable condition will be made a more or less acceptable one to live with.

I am grateful to Prof. Jens J. Pindborg for his valuable comments on the manuscript. Finally, I would like to thank Munksgaard Publishers for their pleasant and correct collaboration.

Isaäc van der Waal

Contents

CHAPTER 1

Introduction and Terminology

Introduction

»In the morning she feels fine, has little or no problem (did not wear the denture during the night), but in the late afternoon it gets worse and at night the burning sensation becomes unbearable. Finally, she takes a tranquillizer and goes to bed. Her mouth tastes very bad and that is why she does not eat very much. I hope I have made things clear and that this may contribute to a better understanding of my mother's problems.«

The quotation is from one of the many rather characteristic letters of patients, in this case the daughter of a patient, who took part in a written inquiry among patients who suffer from the burning mouth syndrome (BMS)[78]. BMS, still further to be defined, indeed seems to embitter life for patients completely. Also family and close friends are often bowed down by the misery of the patient.

As dentists and physicians may not be aware of the symptoms of this relatively rare syndrome, patients may find little response for their complaints. On the contrary, the patient may be left with the feeling that his complaints are not taken seriously. At the same time various treatments are carried out that may not be justified.

Patients with oral complaints may consult not only their dentist or family doctor but also may see a number of medical specialists, such as the otolaryngologist, the dermatologist and the neurologist. Also other health care workers, e.g. dental hygienists, can be involved in treating patients with complaints of BMS.

Hampf described 64 patients with orofacial dysesthesia including 17 patients with BMS[39]. As is shown in Table 1,

TABLE 1. Specialists seen by patients with BMS
(n = 17, Hampf [39])

Internist	8
Neurologist	6
Dermatologist	6
Otologist	5
Oral surgeon	4
Allergist	4
Gynaecologist	4
Psychiatrist	3
Ophthalmologist	3
Total	43

the number of specialists consulted, apart from the dentist and family doctor, averaged 2.5 per patient. All patients had already received a number of unsuccessful treatments for their complaints. Those treatments varied from drug prescriptions, extractions of teeth and endodontic treatment to psychiatric treatment. Hampf noted that several patients went through irreversible surgical procedures.

Terminology

In view of the differences in usage among the various dental and medical disciplines, uniformity in terminology will improve the understanding of the problems by the profession and, above all, by the patient.

The terms *glossodynia* or *glossalgia* can be used to describe a painful tongue, and the term *glossopyrosis* to describe a burning sensation in the tongue. When just discomfort is experienced, the term *lingual dysesthesia* can be used. Likewise, for complaints elsewhere in the oral cavity, outside the tongue, the terms *stomatodynia, stomatopyrosis,* and *oral dysesthesia* could be used respectively. For practical reasons, however, the use of the term *burning mouth* is recommended, irrespective of the specific site and nature of the complaint.

10

It is well recognized that many patients complaining of a burning mouth also suffer from a dry mouth, xerostomia, with or without an associated loss of taste or an altered taste sensation, and with or without a number of other symptoms justifying the term *burning mouth syndrome (BMS)*, that will be used in this text.

In denture-wearing patients symptomatic, inflammatory changes that can be observed clinically may occur in the oral mucosa underneath the denture, especially the upper denture. This phenomenon is referred to as *denture stomatitis* or *stomatitis prothetica*[100]. In this condition the symptoms usually regress or disappear completely after removal of the denture. It has been shown that the microflora (especially Candida albicans) of the palatal mucosa and perhaps also of the inner surface of the denture plays a part in the pathogenesis of this condition, which must be clearly separated from BMS.

Denture-wearing patients may occasionally complain of a burning or itching sensation in the mucosa underneath their denture – again especially the upper denture – without clinically observable signs of inflammation. In some of these patients the burning or itching sensation is also experienced in other sites of the oral cavity, e.g. the tongue or the lips. This condition is termed *denture sore mouth* (DSM). In most instances the removal of the dentures does not result in the disappearance of the symptoms. Apparently, there is an overlap between BMS and DSM.

Some authors classify the BMS under the heading of *atypical facial pain* (AFP). AFP, atypical odontalgia[14] and oral dysesthesia, including BMS, may occur sequentially or simultaneously in the same patient, and may be associated with *facial arthromyalgia* in which the temporomandibular joint or its musculature are involved[24].

As will be discussed later in more detail, a distinction is usually made between complaints for which an organic cause can be detected and complaints of unknown, idiopathic etiology. Preferably, the term BMS should be used only in patients with idiopathic complaints.

In conclusion, it is advised for the sake of clarity for

both the patient and the clinician that the term *burning mouth syndrome* be used only in idiopathic cases in which the main symptoms, being described as a burning, painful or itching sensation, are located in the oral mucosa, with or without involvement of the tongue and with or without associated symptoms in the oral cavity or elsewhere in the body.

CHAPTER 2

Epidemiology

There are hardly any epidemiologic data available on the prevalence of BMS in different parts of the world. In most studies the findings in a selected patient population are reported, such as in patients from a general dental practice, or patients visiting a menopause clinic or a diabetic clinic.

General dental practice population

In a study in Birmingham (UK) questionnaires were distributed to five dental practices, to be completed by adult patients who remained anonymous[7]. Replies were received from 392 patients. A prolonged burning sensation had been experienced at some time by more than 5% of the population. The complaint was reported by 4.2% of women and 0.8% of men. A chi-square test revealed that those different percentages were not statistically significant. However, when studying various age groups the sex difference was shown statistically significant in the 40-49 age group ($p < 0.05$) as is shown in Table 2.

TABLE 2. Prevalence of burning according to sex and age of patients participating in a general dental practice survey[7]

	Age group (years)			
	20-29	30-39	40-49	50-59
	%	%	%	%
Men	-	3.2	2.9	3.0
Women	1.5	5.4	15.7	5.4

From the foregoing figures it seems justified to estimate the prevalence of BMS among the adult population at approximately 5%. However, in the study by Basker et al. it was

13

not stated as to how many patients were asked to complete the questionnaires and what percentage of patients refused to do so.

In a survey in the Netherlands the incidence of 26 types of pain in general dental practices was recorded[106]. The results of the 6-week recording in 41 practices – 666 complaints of pain were registered – did not reveal a single case of BMS, although perhaps an occasional patient was included under the heading of neuralgia, which was reported in 6 patients (1%).

In a Danish study on the incidence of pain conditions among patients between 18 and 70 years of age in 30 dental practices, again no BMS patients were reported[90]. Perhaps a few patients were included in the 2% of pain complaints under the heading »others«.

Studies in a menopause clinic

In a group of 114 women attending the Menopause Research Clinic at the Birmingham and Midland Hospital for Women, oral symptoms were reported by 30 patients (26%) who were asked to fill out a self-assessment symptom questionnaire[7]. Of the group of 30 patients with oral symptoms, 43% complained only of burning, 27% of strange tastes and 30% of a combination of both these conditions.

Studies in a diabetic clinic

In a study reported by Basker et al[7] among 110 patients being treated for clinical diabetes, nearly 40% of patients complained of a dry mouth, whereas problems of a burning mouth or abnormal taste were reported in less than 10% of the patients. The total group of 110 patients comprised 49 men and 61 women. No data were provided on the sex ratio of the patients with oral complaints, e.g. burning mouth.

14

Miscellaneous studies

In the majority of papers about BMS the mean age of the patients is around 50-60 years, the range varying considerably. For instance, in the study by Browning et al[16] the youngest patient was 37 and the oldest was 81. In another study of 102 patients the youngest was 36 and the oldest was 84 years old[34].

The reported sex ratio may vary to some extent. In most studies a rather strong female predilection is recorded. In Grushka's study of 102 patients the female:male ratio was about 5:1[34], while in the study reported by Van der Ploeg et al[78] that ratio was as much as 9:1. In a paper on BMS from the Federal Republic of Germany the reported female predilection was less distinct, being just 2.5:1[93]. However, in that paper on 388 patients, 55 patients with lichen planus, 39 patients with denture stomatitis and 12 patients with squamous cell carcinomas of the floor of the mouth and the tongue were included.

In conclusion, it can be stated that no world-wide figures of the prevalence of BMS are available. Therefore, little is known about possible racial and geographic differences in the epidemiologic figures. From the various studies from Europe and North America it can be estimated that BMS probably occurs in 5-10 per 100 000 population. There is a female predilection of more than 3:1. Symptoms of BMS almost exclusively occur in middle-aged and elderly people. Occurrence in patients under the age of 30 years is exceptional.

CHAPTER 3

Symptomatology

Symptoms of BMS

In the introductory chapter it has been explained already that BMS includes a wide variety of complaints. Some patients indeed describe their feelings as having burnt their mouth or tongue (»Hot Tongue Syndrome«) [88], while others complain of prickling, itching or bizarre sensations. Although patients often describe the sensation as being intolerable, it is apparently rarely incapacitating[84]. A somewhat similar experience has been reported by Hughes et al[50], who described the psychiatric disorders seen in 138 consecutive attenders at a psychiatric clinic in a dental hospital. In that group, a large number of BMS patients was included.

The symptoms of BMS almost always have a bilateral pattern and, in contrast to symptoms in neurologic disorders, have a non-anatomic distribution.

Specific sites of complaints

Most patients with BMS describe the burning sensation as occurring at more than one site in the mouth. In several reports the tip of the tongue is the most common location. In Table 3 the sites of burning in 154 patients are presented. Notice that, indeed, multiple sites are mentioned by the patients.

In Van der Ploeg et al's series the floor of the mouth was not mentioned as a site of burning, while in the patients reported by Grushka 13% complained of burning in that specific site[34]. In the latter paper the buccal mucosa was not mentioned as a site of burning. On the other hand, burning sensation was reported in the extracutaneous portion of the lips in approximately 20% of cases.

TABLE 3. Sites of burning in 154 patients
(Van der Ploeg et al [78])

Location	%
Tip of the tongue	71
Lateral borders of the tongue	46
Dorsum of the tongue	46
Lips	50
Buccal mucosa	21
Palate	46
Throat	19
Upper denture-bearing tissue	25
Lower denture-bearing tissue	19
Oral cavity and throat	7

Course of symptoms

Almost without exception, the symptoms of BMS are continuously present over a period of months or years, without distinct periods of remission.

The daily pattern of symptoms is constant for each individual patient. For instance, in some patients the burning is present day and night. In most patients with BMS the symptoms are not present on waking but arise and increase in severity as the day progresses, without preventing the patient from falling asleep. Lamb et al[60] refer to the latter type as BMS type 1 and to the former, where symptoms are constantly present, as type 2. Patients with type 3 have symptomfree days [63a].

In Grushka's study of 102 patients with BMS, burning increased with tension, fatigue, speaking and eating in a considerable number of patients[34]. On the other hand, burning abated in about half the patients while eating meals or cold snacks, or while working or distracted. Alcohol reduced the burning in a quarter of Grushka's patients.

Onset of symptoms

In Grushka's study the onset of BMS was related to a previous dental procedure in 33% of the subjects and to a previous illness in 10%, while 57% of the patients could not relate it to any prior event[34]. In Schoenberg's group of 25 patients, 64% related the onset of symptoms to dental procedures, 24% to the death or threatened loss of a loved one, 6% to menopause and 6% to retirement, overt depression or multiple somatic complaints[84]. The findings in Van der Ploeg et al's patients are summarized, together with Grushka's patients and those of Schoenberg, in Table 4.

TABLE 4. Onset of symptoms in BMS (in %)

Event	Feinmann and Harris*[24]	Grushka[34]	Van der Ploeg et al[78]
Dental treatment	?	33	40
Medical treatment or illness	?	10	21
Adverse life events	82	-	33
Unknown	?	57	6

*(incl. psychogenic facial pain)

Of 93 patients with so-called psychogenic facial pain, including a fair number of patients with BMS, 82% had suffered an adverse life event such as family health problems, bereavement, move of house, or marital difficulty prior to the onset of pain[24].

Quantitation of symptoms

In some studies the use of a visual analogue scale (VAS) and graphic rating scales has been reported for quantitation of symptoms such as pain intensity. It has been demonstrated that the intensity of BMS pain is comparable in intensity to toothache[34].

Scott and Huskisson concluded that the VAS and the graphic rating scales used horizontally with the words spread out along the whole length of the line are the most satisfactory ones[85].

Graphic rating scale (modified after Scott & Huskisson[85])		
burning as bad as it could be	———————————— serveremoderateslight	no pain

In preparing a scale, the following points should be considered:

1. Define the sensation or response to be observed.
2. Decide on the extremes of the sensation or response; the end phrases should not be so extremely worded as never to be employed. It is not necessary to alternate the scheme of the scales.
3. The descriptive terms should be short, readily understood expressions.
4. The median of the response should be in the center of the line.
5. Numbers should not be superimposed on a visual analogue scale because certain numbers are preferred and interfere with the distribution of vaults.
6. The line should be of a length that may be grasped as a unit (10 cm is convenient) and should have definite »cut off« points.
7. The scale should be introduced with an appropriate question.

When assessing the response to analgesics, Scott and Huskisson recommend using a pain relief score rather than measuring pain. Feinmann and Harris recorded the severity and frequency of pain on a 0-4 scale:

0 = no pain,
1 = mild, occasional pain,
2 = moderate, frequent pain,
3 = marked, frequent pain,
4 = severe, constant pain[25].

19

Other oral complaints in BMS

Most authors have mentioned a number of other oral complaints in BMS patients. Of 17 patients reported by Hampf, disturbance in taste and olfaction was recorded in 6, while atypical toothache was an accompanying symptom in 1[39]. Xerostomia is among the most commonly reported associated symptoms, being noted in about 50% of Haneke's patients[42], and in more than 60% of the patients reported by Grushka[34]. In the latter report altered taste perception, difficulty in swallowing, other throat problems and altered olfaction were recorded in 35, 28, 21 and 13% respectively (Table 5). The increased percentages of xerostomia and persistent taste were significant at $p < 0.001$, while thirst was significantly more common in BMS patients at $p < 0.05$.

TABLE 5. Prevalence (%) of other oral symptoms associated with BMS (Grushka[34])

	BMS (n=54)	Control group, age and sex-matched (n = 27)
Dry mouth	63	19
Persistent taste	60	7
Altered taste perception	35	7
Thirst	37	10
Difficulty swallowing	28	7
Other throat problems	21	4
Altered olfaction	13	8

Other somatic complaints

In Sharp's group of 86 patients with the so-called hot tongue syndrome, 25 patients complained of gastrointestinal symptoms[88]. Constipation, heartburn, nausea, vomiting and symptoms of colitis were described in that order of frequency.

In a series of 43 patients[24], including an unspecified number of patients with BMS, headaches, migraine, neck/back ache, skin disorders, spastic colon and dysfunctional uterine bleeding were recorded in a large percentage of cases. In another group of 17 patients with glossodynia complaints of gastritis and colitis were mentioned by only 2 patients[39].

Grushka compared the number of chronic pain complaints other than BMS between a group of BMS patients and a control group[34]. The number of persons with at least one chronic pain complaint other than BMS was not significantly higher for the BMS subjects than for the control subjects, but the mean number of chronic pains other than BMS per patient was significantly higher for the BMS group than for the control group.

CHAPTER 4

Local Causes of BMS–Like Symptoms

Mucosal lesions and disorders

Many mucosal lesions and disorders may produce BMS-like symptoms. It is therefore important to discuss those lesions in order to separate true, idiopathic BMS from BMS-like conditions. In some instances BMS-like symptoms are caused by faulty dentures or by dental abnormalities. Allergy, smoking habits, the use of alcohol, and changes in the quality or amount of saliva are among the other often-mentioned causes of BMS that will be discussed in this chapter.

Thorough examination of the oral cavity and particularly of the oral mucosa is mandatory. This requires a good light source. The examination involves both inspection and careful palpation of the oral mucosa. Partial or complete dentures should be removed. In order to carry out a proper examination of the tongue, the patient should be asked to extend it. The examiner can hold the tip of the tongue with a square of gauze and then ask the patient to relax. This will permit an adequate inspection and palpation of the tongue and also of the floor of the mouth.

The taking of biopsies of clinically normal-looking oral mucosa in patients with symptoms of BMS is useless. Histologic examination of the buccal mucosa in 24 BMS patients did not show any abnormality; furthermore, there was no epithelial atrophy[42]. In another German study in 29 patients with BMS, biopsies were taken from the lower lip[67]. The findings were compared with 12 postmortem biopsies. In BMS patients, fewer acini were present while an intense infiltrate of lymphocytes and plasma cells was present. The significance of these findings remains somewhat unclear. No other similar studies have been reported. For more detailed information on the lesions to be discussed in this chapter, the reader is referred to one of the standard works in this field by Pindborg[76].

Candidiasis

Candidiasis, also called moniliasis, is a lesion or a group of lesions caused by the fungus Candida albicans, which belongs to the subfamily Cryptococcoideae. In about one quarter of the population the presence of Candida albicans can be shown in the oral flora. Candida is more often found in women than in men. In BMS patients Candida species, and also coliforms, seem to be more prevalent than in healthy individuals [83a].

The growth of Candida can be stimulated by several local and general factors, resulting in penetration into the upper layers of the epithelium. Local predisposing factors are chronic irritation, poor oral hygiene and hyposalivation. The role of smoking in the etiology of candidiasis is questionable. Endocrine disturbances, malnutrition, malabsorption, radiotherapy and the use of corticosteroids and cytostatic drugs are the most common systemic factors that seem to promote the development of candidiasis. And now, infection with the human immunodeficiency virus has been shown to be another important predisposing factor.

It is possible that Candida albicans plays a part in the etiology of glossitis rhombica mediana, which will be discussed later. A specific form of candidiasis, which will not be dealt with here, is so-called angular cheilitis of the commissures, also called »perleches«.

Candidiasis may be classified into pseudomembranous, erythematous or atrophic, and into plaque or nodular types. There is also a type involving the skin and the nails, referred to as chronic mucocutaneous candidiasis (CMCC). In the pseudomembranous type white, slightly elevated plaques that have a milky aspect and that can be rubbed off can be seen. This type mainly occurs on the cheek mu-

23

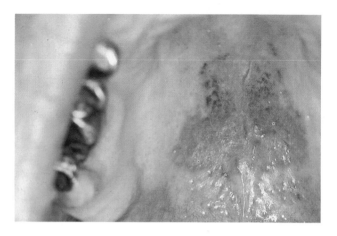

Fig. 1. Candidiasis (erythematous type) of the palatal mucosa.

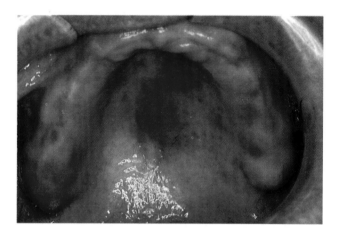

Fig. 2. Erythematous candidiasis (»denture stomatitis«).

cosa and the palate. The erythematous type of candidiasis is manifested by flat, red changes of the mucosa and especially affects the dorsum of the tongue and the palate (Fig. 1). The plaque and the nodular types are characterized by white, sometimes slightly raised changes in the mucosa and mainly occur in the commissures, the dorsum of the tongue and the palate.

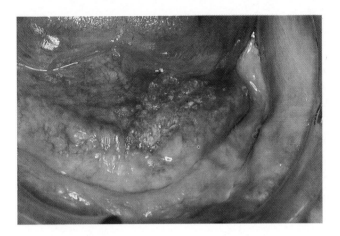

Fig. 3. Subtle changes of the floor of the mouth (left side) caused by a squamous cell carcinoma.

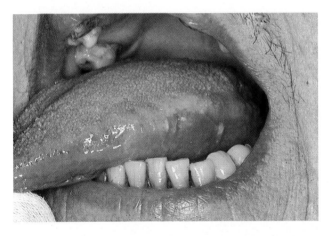

Fig. 4. An elderly woman complained of a burning sensation at the border of the tongue. No biopsy was taken (see Fig. 5).

Especially the erythematous and the pseudomembranous types may cause symptoms such as a painful or burning sensation and sometimes also general malaise.

Some investigators state that, in patients wearing dentures and suffering from denture stomatitis (see p. 11) one always is dealing with candidiasis of an erythematous or atrophic type (Fig. 2).

25

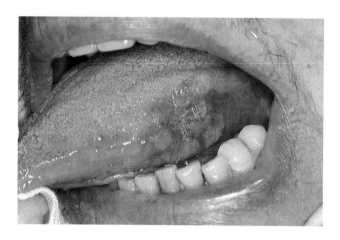

Fig. 5. Same patient as shown in Fig. 4. Almost a year later a squamous cell carcinoma was diagnosed.

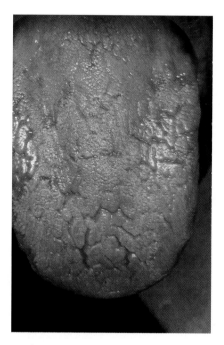

Fig. 6. Fissured tongue may cause a burning or itching sensation.

The presence of Candida can be demonstrated by cytologic examination of the scrapings of the mucosal surface. The scrapings are treated with 20% potassium hydroxide (KOH), after which the candidal hyphae, if present,

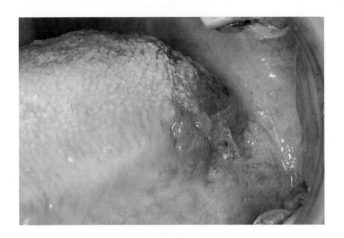

Fig. 7. Foliate papillitis, left side (see Fig. 8).

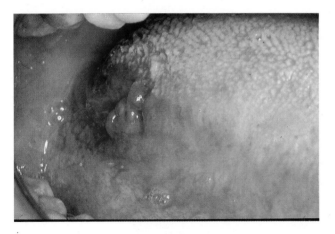

Fig. 8. Same patient as shown in Fig. 7. Foliate papillitis, right side.

become clearly visible. Further identification of the micro-organisms is obtained by culturing, e.g., in a blood agar medium. Some investigators quantify the results of the culturing using grades like 2+, 3+ etc.

When a biopsy specimen is available the presence of candidal hyphae in the superficial part of the epithelium is best demonstrated by the use of a periodic acid-Schiff

27

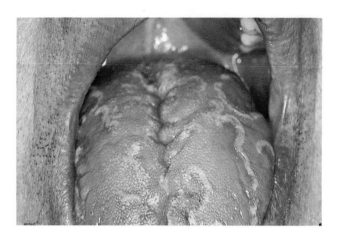

Fig. 9. Well recognizable pattern of geographic tongue.

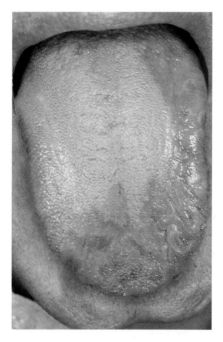

Fig. 10. Less obvious, but definitely present pattern of geographic tongue.

(PAS) stain. The other histologic features vary, depending on the particular type of candidiasis. In some cases rather characteristic microabscesses in the surface layers of the epithelium can be observed. Usually, there is a nonspecific

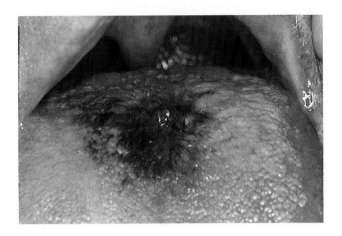

Fig. 11. Hairy tongue.

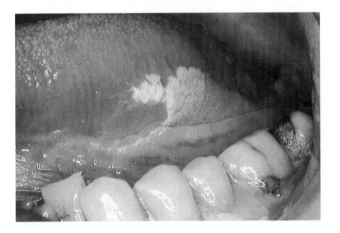

Fig. 12. Leukoplakia of the tongue, homogeneous type.

lymphoplasmacellular infiltrate present in the lamina propria and the subepithelial connective tissue.

In daily practice the diagnosis is often based on the results of antifungal treatment without preceding cytologic or histologic examination.

Treatment of candidiasis consists of mouth rinses and/or local application of antifungal drugs such as Nystatin®, 29

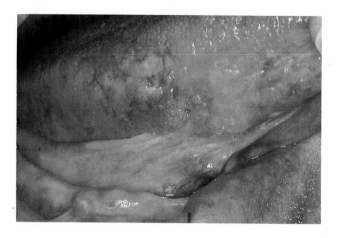

Fig. 13. Leukoplakia of the tongue, non-homogeneous type.

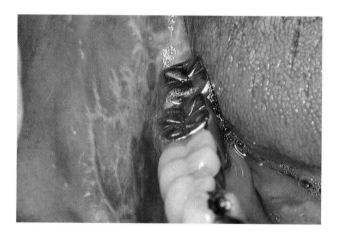

Fig. 14. Lichen planus of cheek mucosa, reticular type.

100 000 units per g x 3 a day, with or without 10 mg am-photericin-B lozenges of 10 mg x 4 a day. Such a regimen can be continued for a few weeks without a risk of harm-ful side-effects. The effect of treatment is often limited to the time during which the drug is used[22]. In rare cases, Nystatine resistance necessitates the use of a different drug. Of course, possible predisposing factors such as

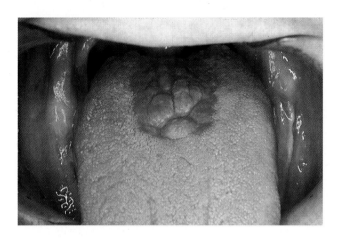

Fig. 15. Median rhomboid glossitis.

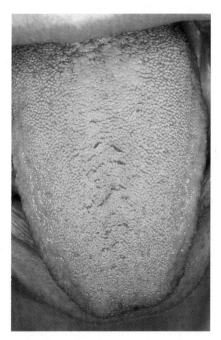

Fig. 16. Apparently normal aspect of the tongue in a patient suffering from BMS. The symptoms were mainly localized in the tongue.

smoking or an incorrect vertical dimension of dentures should be eliminated first.

In 15 patients with BMS who had no clinical symptoms of candidiasis and whose number of positive culturings of

31

Candida albicans corresponded with that of the general population, an improvement of the complaints was obtained in 86% of the patients using antifungal lozenges; in 13% the complaints completely disappeared [32]. One should realize, however, that the number of patients was rather small. Besides, the results were not based on a double-blind examination. One may actually have been dealing with a so-called placebo effect. In fact, antifungal drugs seem to be used quite often as a panacea in a wide variety of oral complaints, leaving the patient with the impression that he or she is suffering from a fungal disease.

Carcinoma

A carcinoma is a malignant neoplasm of epithelial origin.

About 3% of all malignant diseases occurring in the body arise in the oral cavity. The majority consists of carcinomas derived from the mucosa. Squamous cell carcinomas most often affect middle-aged and elderly people. In many parts of the world there is a strong predilection for men, but this is less distinct in Europe and North America.

The excessive use of tobacco, especially when combined with heavy consumption of alcohol, is an important factor in the etiology of oral cancer. Other factors that may play a role as promoting factors are chronic mechanic irritation by a poor dentition or an ill-fitting denture and poor oral hygiene. Especially in elderly women, often none of the above-mentioned etiologic factors is present.

The symptoms of oral carcinomas vary widely. Especially in early carcinomas of the tongue and the floor of the mouth, burning or itching may be the first sign. In these instances the symptoms are localized at a specific site, which is different from the symptoms in BMS (Figs. 3 and 4).

Oral carcinomas usually present themselves as an indurated ulcer. A submucosal swelling or an exophytic, verrucous appearance is less common. Occasionally, the first mucosal changes that are indicative of malignancy consist of leukoplakic or erythroplakic changes, with or without induration (Fig. 5).

Sites of predilection are the borders of the tongue, the floor of the mouth and, to a lesser extent, the mucosa of the alveolar ridges, the cheek mucosa and the lower lip.

A diagnosis of squamous cell carcinoma should always be based on the histologic findings of a biopsy.

It is beyond the scope of this text to discuss the various aspects of treatment.

Erythroplakia

The term erythroplakia is used analogously to leukoplakia to designate a lesion of the oral mucosa that appears as a bright red patch or plaque that can not be characterized clinically or pathologically as any other disease.

In most instances the lesion is fiery red and well demarcated. In some patients leukoplakic changes can be seen intermingled with the lesion, making it an erythroleukoplakia or just a non-homogeneous leukoplakia.

Erythroplakia usually causes symptoms of a localized burning sensation or just an unpleasant irritation.

There will always be dysplasia or carcinoma in an erythroplakia. Therefore, treatment is required.

Fissured tongue

Fissured tongue, also called plicated or scrotal tongue, represents a clinically visible change in the dorsal surface of the anterior two-thirds of the tongue. Several definitions have been suggested, such as »a tongue with or without a central fissure which shows parallel fissures at right angles to the long axis of the tongue«, or, »a tongue characterized by furrows, one extending anteroposteriorly and others laterally over the entire surface«.

The etiology of fissured tongue is unknown, although a developmental nature seems most likely. In an unselected Swedish adult population, a prevalence of 7% was reported by Axell[3]. The condition is found more frequently in the elderly[12]. There is no sex predilection.

33

The fissures may be relatively shallow or may be deep, in which case food debris will accumulate (Fig. 6). In 20% of patients with fissured tongue the simultaneous presence of geographic tongue is observed [19].

Most patients with fissured tongue are not aware of the condition. Only in rare instances is some discomfort experienced, being quite different from the symptoms of BMS, both with regard to the duration and the intensity.

In case of discomfort the patient may be advised to carefully brush the tongue a few times a day with lukewarm water.

Foliate papillitis

Foliate papillae can be described as projections arranged in folds along the posterolateral border of the tongue. The folds are separated by grooves of different depths perpendicular to the longitudinal axis of the tongue [96].

The subepithelial connective tissue of a foliate papilla contains a variable number of lymphocytes and sometimes a lymph follicle, making the distinction from a lingual tonsil difficult [91]. Hypertrophy of lymphoid tissue may be followed by secondary traumatization, resulting in so-called foliate papillitis. Clinically, an area of redness may be observed (Figs. 7 and 8).

Symptoms may consist of unilateral or bilateral tenderness or pain [87]. In case of unilateral symptoms the main concern is to rule out the possibility of a squamous cell carcinoma. This usually requires the taking of a biopsy. In case of bilateral occurrence the symptoms may mimic those of BMS to some extent. However, in the case of BMS the symptoms are of a more diffuse nature and are, in most instances, located in other oral sites as well.

Treatment of foliate papillitis can only consist of elimination of irritating factors such as sharp edges of teeth or dentures.

Fuso-spirochetal infection

In a study by Katz et al [57] 6 middle-aged and elderly edentulous patients,complaining of burning sensations in the
mouth, particularly the tongue, have been described. The
medical histories revealed that the patients suffered from
chronic illnesses, such as lupus erythematodes, glomeru-
lonephritis, rheumatoid arthritis and diabetes mellitus. In
all patients the presence of a coated tongue was mentioned.

Direct smears taken from the tongue, stained with
Giemsa, showed spirochetes and fusiform bacteria. Improvement in all patients was reported after the use of te-
tracycline mouthwash (250 mg/5ml water x 4 daily for 1
week). Three patients were additionally treated with me-
tronidazole (250 mg x 3 daily for 1 week), resulting in a
complete disappearence of the burning complaints. One
year later the patients were reportedly free of symptoms.
The authors recommended that smears be taken routinely
to search for the presence of fusospirochetes in patients
suffering from BMS.

No similar experiences have since been reported in the
literature.

Geographic tongue

Geographic tongue, also referred to as erythema migrans,
is a benign condition of unknown etiology characterized
by the occurrence of one or more smooth areas on the
dorsum and the lateral borders of the tongue (Figs. 9 and
10). In the smooth areas there is an absence of filiform papillae. Similar lesions may occur elsewhere on the oral
mucosa, and these are referred to as geographic stomatitis [52].

The prevalence can be estimated at at least 1% to 2%,
without a distinct preference for race, sex or age [6].

Infection, emotional disturbances, allergy, and heredity
are among the most commonly suggested etiologic factors.
The often simultaneous occurrence of geographic tongue

35

and fissured tongue is well known and is possibly due to a common genetic factor.

A geographic tongue is often asymptomatic and many patients are, indeed, not aware of the condition. Some patients, however, may experience BMS-like symptoms. In contrast with BMS, the symptoms of geographic tongue are related to the consumption of food and drinks, and the site of the symptoms correlates well with the clinically visible changes of the lingual mucosa. In a number of papers on BMS patients the presence of geographic tongue has been mentioned. Gorsky et al[32] noticed this in as many as 15% of their patients.

The diagnosis of geographic tongue rarely needs histopathologic confirmation. The microscopic appearance is characterized by numerous polymorphonuclear leukocytes that migrate through the epithelium and give rise to the formation of small abscesses. The stratum spinosum may be thickened and edematous. In the smooth, red areas the papillae of the connective tissue may reach high up, close to the surface.

Almost no effective treatments or preventive measures are available. In a Swedish study the successful use of local application of a solution of 7% salicylic acid in 70% alcohol has been reported[47]. Good results have also been claimed with the topical use of 0.1% tretinoin[46].

Hairy tongue

Hairy tongue, or lingua villosa, designates an overgrowth of the filiform papillae of the dorsum of the tongue, giving the tongue a superficial appearance of hairiness.

In an adult population the prevalence is in the range of 0.5% to 1%. The cause of hairy tongue is not well understood. Possible causes are the use of hydrogen peroxide, topical application of antibiotics, poor oral hygiene, and heavy smoking.

The affected papillae are usually located in the posterior part of the dorsal surface. The color of hairy tongue may vary from white to yellow, from gray to brown and black (Fig. 11). The pigmentation is thought to be the result of tobacco, impaction of food, or overgrowth of chromogenic microorganisms.

Hairy tongue may be asymptomatic. In extensive cases, discomfort or an itching sensation is experienced either locally on the tongue itself or on the palate, mimicking BMS symptoms to some extent. No biopsy is required to establish the diagnosis.

Hairy tongue may disappear spontaneously in a matter of weeks, but may also persist for years. Brushing the tongue twice daily for 2 minutes with water, making gentle movements over the involved area toward the tip of the tongue, may give excellent results in a matter of days.

Leukoplakia

Leukoplakia is defined as a white patch on the oral mucosa that cannot be characterized clinically or pathologically as any other diagnosable disease and is not associated with any physical or chemical causative agent except tobacco[4].

Leukoplakia is considered a premalignant lesion. Of all oral leukoplakias about 5% will develop into a squamous cell carcinoma within an average of 5 years.

Leukoplakic changes occur particularly after age 30. There is a distinct preference for the male sex. Chronic irritation, either from a sharp edge of a tooth or a denture, or from overuse of tobacco, is considered the main cause of leukoplakia. In leukoplakic lesions, the presence of Candida albicans can often be demonstrated. Whether that microorganism is a true causative factor in the etiology of leukoplakia or simply a secondary phenomenon has yet to be established.

Sites of preference are the cheek mucosa, the commissures and to a lesser extent the borders of the tongue, the floor of the mouth, and the lower lip. In general, two clinical types of oral leukoplakia are recognized, a homogene-

37

ous and a non-homogeneous type (Figs. 12 and 13). The latter type can be further subdivided into erythroleukoplakia, erosive, nodular, and verrucous leukoplakia.

Symptoms are usually only present in the non-homogeneous types and may consist of burning or itching sensations, mimicking to some extent the symptoms of BMS. However, symptoms related to leukoplakia are localized and correspond with clinically visible changes of the mucosa.

Leukoplakia should not be diagnosed solely on the basis of clinical judgement, without taking a biopsy, particularly in the case of localization on the tongue and the floor of the mouth.

The histologic aspects of leukoplakia may vary from hyperkeratosis, with or without epithelial dysplasia, to carcinoma in situ and even squamous cell carcinoma.

Treatment very much depends on the histologic findings of the biopsy and the possible etiologic factor(s). For instance, the complete cessation of smoking may cause some leukoplakias to disappear completely after a few months. When the removal of leukoplakia is indicated, surgical excision is still the treatment of choice, since it enables reliable histopathologic examination of the surgical specimen.

Continuous follow-up is indicated for any patient with oral leukoplakia, whether or not it is being treated. The time interval may vary from 3 to 6 months.

Lichen planus

Lichen planus is an inflammatory disease of the skin and mucous membranes with a typical clinical papular appearance accompanied by characteristic Wickham's striae.

The cause is unknown. A number of possible agents have been suggested, such as fungi, viruses, trauma, stress, galvanism, and immunological disturbance. In recent years emphasis has been placed on the possibility of contact allergy to dental materials such as amalgam[69]. Lichenoid reactions have also been described as resulting from the use of certain drugs. In a study from Sweden of a group of 40 patients with oral lichen planus, a significant number of patients with diabetes mellitus was recorded[68].

Epidemiologic surveys of oral lichen planus are rare. A study of 20 333 individuals showed a prevalence rate of 1.9%, with a significantly higher rate for women than for men[3].

Oral lichen planus may assume a variety of morphologic changes, such as papular, reticular, plaque-like, atrophic, ulcerative, erosive, and bullous (Fig. 14).

The cheek mucosa and to a lesser degree the tongue and the gums are the sites of predilection. In the majority of patients multiple, more or less symmetrical lesions are present.

Lichen planus of the oral mucosa, in particular the erosive type, is sometimes accompanied by a painful, burning sensation. The symptoms are often of an intermittent nature and correspond with the clinically visible mucosal changes, which is quite different from the symptoms in idiopathic BMS.

In many cases the diagnosis of lichen planus can be made based on the clinical appearance, making a biopsy superfluous.

The different types of oral lichen planus lesions exhibit variations in histologic appearance. The papular, reticular, and plaque-like types are characterized by a marked hyperorthokeratosis or hyperparakeratosis with a broad granular cell layer. The presence of liquefaction degeneration of the basal epithelial layer and a band-like juxtaepithelial infiltrate dominated by lymphocytes are noted in all types.

Treatment of oral lichen planus can only be symptomatic. Because of the secondary presence of Candida albicans in some cases, the use of fungicides may produce considerable improvement. The patients may also benefit from the local application of corticosteroids, e.g. Kenacortinorabase® or Topsyne®. In case of more severe complaints, triamcinolone acetonide, 10 mg per 1 ml can be injected intralesionally, 0.1 ml per 1 square cm. Such in-

jections can be repeated weekly. A 50% mixture with lidocaine can be used to reduce the pain of the injection.

Median rhomboid glossitis

Median rhomboid glossitis (MRG) is a benign lesion of the
tongue characterized by rhomboid or oval-shaped
changes of the mucosa in the dorsal midline just anteriorly
to the foramen cecum.

The prevalence varies from 0.28% to 1.39%. There is no
preference for race or sex. The diagnosis is most often
made in middle-aged patients.

The etiology is not well understood. Most authors today
stress the possible role of Candida albicans either as a primary invader or as a secondary phenomenon. Actually,
MRG should perhaps be regarded as an erythematous type
of candidiasis. Defective immunity may act as a promoting
factor, since MRG-like changes are often observed in HIV-
seropositive patients. The role of smoking as a causative or
promoting factor is questionable.

Clinically, MRG is characterized by a flat or slightly elevated and in some cases lobulated lesion located just anteriorly to the foramen cecum (Fig. 15). The lesion may be
rhomboid or oval-shaped, usually varies in size from 1 to 2
cm, and is rather well-demarcated. The texture may vary
from a reddish smooth or granular surface to a more lobulated and indurated aspect. Although there may be some
resemblance to the clinical picture of a squamous cell carcinoma, it should be realized that such a tumor rarely, if
ever, arises at this particular site of the tongue. In some patients with MRG somewhat similar changes on the oppo-
site palatal mucosa can be observed.

Most patients are asymptomatic and are unaware of
their lingual lesion. Some patients, however, complain of
slight discomfort, being described as burning or itching.

The diagnosis of MRG can almost always be made by
clinical judgment. Cultures, cytologic scrapings, or biopsy
specimens show the presence of Candida albicans in the
majority of cases.

Treatment, if necessary, consists of withdrawal of smoking habits and the local application of fungicides.

Stomatitis

Stomatitis refers to an erythematous change in part or all of the oral and lingual mucosa, presumably being of a reactive nature. When the gingiva is involved, the term gingivostomatitis is used. Stomatitis is usually extremely painful and the symptoms are often described as a burning sensation. Depending on the underlying cause, symptoms of general malaise may be present. The etiology is quite diverse. For instance, herpes simplex virus can be involved, referred to as herpetiform stomatitis. Also the possibility of infection with the human immunodeficiency virus should be mentioned here. With scarlet fever there is the so-called stomatitis scarlatina. Although relatively rare, gonococcal infection may be another cause of stomatitis.

Stomatitis nicotina is a rather peculiar type of stomatitis that is more or less limited to the palate and is caused by smoking habits, especially by pipe-smoking, and therefore is also referred to as smoker's palate.

In rare instances stomatitis can be the sign and symptom of an underlying blood disorder, e.g. agranulocytosis, cyclic neutropenia and various types of leukemia.

In the introductory chapter the terms denture stomatitis and stomatitis prothetica have been mentioned already. These terms refer to clinically observable red, and sometimes hyperplastic changes of the mucosa underneath a denture, in almost all cases the upper denture (Fig. 2). Many studies have related Candida albicans to this type of stomatitis. Poor oral and denture hygiene seems an important predisposing factor.

Radiotherapy can be another cause or predisposing factor in stomatitis.

Possibilities for treatment largely depend on the causative factor(s).

41

Dentures as primary cause

Introduction

BMS is definitely not limited to patients wearing partial or full dentures. In a group of 55 patients who were not suffering from mucosal lesions and in whom no systemic or neurologic cause of their symptoms could be detected, 36% had a natural dentition[78]. This finding strongly argues against the hypothesis that dentures are the main cause of BMS.

As has been explained in the introductory chapter, a distinction should be made between BMS and denture stomatitis (stomatitis prothetica) and also between BMS and denture sore mouth (see p. 11).

Faulty dentures

In a series of 37 patients complaining of a burning mouth, denture faults (occlusion, articulation, stability etc.) were considered the single most tangible cause in 50%[70]. In patients whose symptoms were closely related to the wearing of dentures 100% were shown to have faulty dentures while less than half had some other cause. In patients whose symptoms were not related to the wearing of dentures, faulty dentures were present in only 30% while 95% were found to have a non-denture cause. When there was an association of burning symptoms with the wearing of dentures, the site of burning in the majority of cases was the denture-bearing tissues, whereas when non-association was recorded the more common sites of burning were in other areas of the oral mucosa. Apparently, in almost all patients complete resolution of symptoms, or at least considerable improvement, was obtained after elimination of the causitive factors, including those related to the dentures.

42 In Main and Basker's paper the criteria for faulty den-

tures were not specified[70]. Furthermore, it is not clear from their paper whether or not clinically visible changes were present in the denture-bearing mucosa in the patients whose symptoms were related to the wearing of dentures. In other words, one may have been dealing both with patients with denture stomatitis and with patients with denture sore mouth.

In a group of 22 patients complaining of a burning sensation related to denture wearing, faults in stability, fit or occlusion were found in 12 of them[1]. However, the burning mouth sensation persisted in 11 cases following correction of the denture faults which were thought to be etiologically significant. Moreover, in an age- and sex-matched control group of healthy denture wearers without signs or symptoms, 86% had denture faults, questioning the significance of such faults with regard to BMS-like symptoms.

Sensitivity to acrylic resin

The significance of sensitizing compound in the denture base for the etiology of BMS has been studied in 53 denture-wearing patients[56]. The symptoms consisted of intermittent, but intense sensations of dryness, soreness or burning in the denture contact area and the adjacent oral regions, predominantly the tongue and the lip mucosa. Patch tests were performed on the skin of the back, using a standard series of various sensitizing compounds known to be present in denture base materials (Table 6).

In 14 of the 53 cases patch testing showed positive skin reaction to one or more of the compounds used as allergens. In 11 of these cases the positive skin reactions had its oral counterpart in inflammatory mucosal changes, which ranged from distinct erythema to a generalized fiery-red surface accompanied by edema in the adjacent soft tissue. Apparently, these patients were suffering from denture stomatitis. In the remaining 3 cases the denture-bearing mucosa showed no obvious inflammatory changes, ranging from a clinically normal texture to an atrophic appear-

43

TABLE 6. Potential sensitizing compounds in denture base material (Kaaber et al [56])

Test substance	Patch test concentration(%) and vehicle	
Methylmethacrylate	30	olive oil
Hydroquinone	1	1 petrolatum
Benzoyl peroxide	1	1 pet
Dimethyl-p-toluidine	30	olive oil
Dibutyl phthalate	5	pet
p-phenylendiamine	1	pet
Formaldehyde	2	aqueous sol.
Cadmium sulfate	2	pet
Potassium dichromate	0.5	pet
Cobalt chloride	1	pet
Nickel sulfate	5	pet
Filings from own denture		saliva

ance, yet without erythema. These are the patients with denture sore mouth. The construction of new dentures using alternative materials resulted in partial or total relief of the symptoms. In a similar study reported by Wakkers-Garritsen et al [105], none of the 23 patients showed positive skin reactions. The reason for this discrepancy is unclear.

In a study of 22 patients complaining of a burning mouth sensation related to denture wearing, 5 were found by skin patch testing to be allergic to methyl methacrylate monomer in their acrylic dentures[1]. All these patients had high residual monomer levels in their dentures, ranging from 0.35% to 2.0%. In 2 of the 5 patients replacement acrylic dentures with low residual monomer had no effect on the symptoms. Interestingly, 50% of control subjects had high residual monomer levels without any signs or symptoms, making this subject far from understood.

McCabe and Basker[71] described a chromatographic

technique for determining the percentage of residual monomer in acrylic dentures. This method has been applied in patients in whom the denture base, although heat-cured, had been incorrectly processed, resulting in high levels of residual monomer.

From the foregoing studies it can be concluded that patch testing and determination of residual monomer levels in symptomatic denture-wearing patients is only indicated in the presence of stomatitis. This view is also shared by some other authors[8].

Odontogenic causes

Dental treatment

As has been mentioned before, dental treatment is considered the main and only cause of the symptoms of BMS by a large proportion of patients (see p. 18). This applies to all types of dental treatment procedures, including root canal treatment and extraction of teeth. On the other hand, patients with BMS are often convinced that a certain type of dental treatment will eliminate their symptoms and desperately ask for extraction of one or more, or even of all teeth. Already in 1924 Frazier et al recommended abstinence from active dental or oral surgical treatment in patients with atypical facial pain, including BMS, if no specific indication for such treatment was present. In a more recent study it was shown that, in about 75% of patients suffering from atypical facial pain, different types of treatment such as extractions of teeth and endodontic treatment had been instituted in a vain attempt to alleviate the pain, often aggravating the symptoms[73]. In some of those cases cessation of active treatment noticeably reduced the symptoms. In yet another study, 21 of 58 patients (36%) with atypical facial pain had 65 dental and surgical treatments, with only 1 patient showing less pain as a result of the treatment[82].

45

Galvanism

Oral galvanism refers to the phenomenon of currents resulting from an electrochemical reaction between dissimilar dental metallic restorations in the presence of a conducting solution such as saliva. The magnitude of currents can be calculated after measurements of potentials and polarizations of metallic restorations [10].

The attributed complaints are often described as being of a smarting or burning sensation. A metallic taste is another, rather common complaint. Although it has been suggested that galvanism can be the cause of mucosal lesions, no scientifically proven data are available to substantiate that hypothesis. Papers on this subject had been published already in 1932 [48].

In a group of patients referred with symptoms presumably related to oral galvanism, a broad spectrum of local and systemic symptoms was recorded [5]. Strikingly, there was a strong similarity with the symptoms in patients suffering from BMS. Also the commonly reported distinct female predilection in BMS patients was noticed. When comparing the findings in these patients with those of a control group regarding to the calculated maximum current at the contact between metallic restorations, no statistically significant differences could be detected.

In another study from Sweden, comprising 62 patients referred because of presumed galvanism, a complex symptomatology was observed [55]. Symptoms from both the oral regions and other parts of the body constituted the most distinctive features of the patients in the test group, compared with a sex- and age-matched control group without symptoms. The findings at the oral and medical examination revealed no differences between the groups, except for signs of parafunction which were significantly more prevalent among the test group.

In yet another group of 100 patients referred for the investigation of complaints related to oral galvanism, oral, dental and medical explanations for the symptoms could be given in most cases [51]. Only in a very few patients could the symptoms and the clinical diagnosis be attributed to dental restorative materials.

Metal allergy

Metal alloys that are used in restorative dentistry contain ions of gold, paladium, zinc, molybdenum, tin, gallium, indium, cobalt, chrome, nickel, iron and silicon. Using patch tests on the skin, three groups of patients were examined for possible hypersensitivity to one or more of the aforementioned metal ions[66]. Group 1 consisted of patients with a positive history of contact stomatitis. Group 2 consisted of patients with a positive history of contact dermatitis, and group 3 consisted of a control group. In groups 1 and 2 a higher percentage of patients showed a positive skin reaction to one or more of the test metals compared with the control group. The differences were most evident in reactions to paladium and nickel. It was striking that, in group 1 13% of the patients showed a positive reaction for gold.

The significance of the aforementioned findings with regard to symptoms of BMS is not completely clear. But the study showed that, in a more or less objective way, any hypersensitivity for materials used in restorative dentistry can be detected. Whether or not the elimination of such materials truly influences the symptoms of BMS remains to be proven.

Malocclusion

The role of malocclusion of the upper and lower dental arches does not seem to be of major importance in the etiology of BMS. The same applies to malpositioning of teeth and the presence of clasps of partial dentures.

Oral hygiene

The hypothesis that poor oral hygiene can cause a burning 47 sensation, or can aggravate existing complaints, has never been proven.

Food allergy

In many BMS patients the use of spicy food will worsen the symptoms of burning. This should not be interpreted as being the result of an allergic reaction, but seems merely to be the result of local irritation. The same applies to certain drinks, such as orange juice or sparkling white wine. Only in exceptional cases may there be a true allergy, for instance for peppermint oil, chewing gum, toothpaste, mouthrinses and lipstick.

Smoking and the use of alcohol

In a German study in 72 BMS patients, the use of tobacco and alcohol was registered[43] (Table 7).

TABLE 7. The use of tobacco and alcohol in 72 BMS patients (Haneke[43])

Use of tobacco	%	Use of alcohol	%
smoking	15.3	moderate	52.8
heavy smoking	5.5	abuse	1.4

Fifty-five patients in the hospital of the Free University, Amsterdam, were asked to register the usage of alcohol. The results were almost identical to those of the German study (Table 8).

In a group of 98 BMS patients, 34 were smokers[32]. A similar number was found in the general population, which does not support the view that smoking plays an important role in the etiology of BMS. Moreover, the aforementioned study showed that tobacco abstinence did not affect the symptoms.

TABLE 8. The use of alcohol in 55 BMS patients
Free University, Amsterdam

No alcohol	3%
Incidentally (1-2 consumptions a week)	34%
Moderate (3-10 consumptions a week)	47%
Much (more than 10 consumptions a week)	6%
Not clearly stated	9%

Notwithstanding above-mentioned opinion, patients themselves sometimes relate that smoking aggravates the symptoms. The same experience applies to the use of alcohol. On the other hand, as mentioned on p. 17, alcohol may also reduce the symptoms of burning in a fair number of patients.

CHAPTER 5

Systemic Causes

Hormonal disturbances

The rather strong predilection of BMS in menopausal and postmenopausal women is suggestive of a possible hormonal disturbance. However, that hypothesis has never been proven scientifically.

In a group of 114 women visiting a menopause clinic, 26% experienced oral symptoms [7]. In only one-third of the patients did the oral symptoms consist of a burning sensation. Almost all women with menopausal complaints were treated with estrogen and progesterone. In most patients an enormous improvement was seen in the general complaints, such as »hot flushes«, while only a limited improvement was obtained in the oral complaints.

Glick et al [29] examined 50 patients with the complaint of a sore tongue; 26 patients did not have any visible mucosal changes. In this last group, half the patients showed abnormal blood values and were excluded from the study. In the remaining group of 13 patients who were all postmenopausal women, total mixed saliva was collected and compared with the findings in a control group of 13 postmenopausal women with no complaints of a sore tongue. The salivary flow rate was similar in both groups. However, a change in salivary content was found: potassium, protein and phosphate concentrations were significantly higher in the test group than in the control group. Especially the increased concentration of phosphates was interpreted as being a reflection of changes in hormonal balance (see also p. 56).

An interesting study has been performed in a group of 145 women who had been oophorectomized for non-malignant disease [26]. The mean age at the time of the operation for this group was 43.1 years. Apart from the general climacteric symptoms, these 145 women were assessed for oral symptom, and gave their consent to be admitted into a double-blind controlled trial. For a period of 1 year half of the group was given estrogen replacement and the other half was given a placebo. The estrogen group showed a significant improvement of taste disturbance. However, no differences were recorded with regard to the symptoms of dry mouth or a burning sensation (Table 9).

TABLE 9. Comparison of the prevalence of oral symptoms in women treated with placebo or oestrogen (Ferguson et al[26])

	Placebo (n = 71) %	Oestrogen (n = 74) %	Signifi- cance
Unpleasant taste	27.4	15.9	p<0.1
Dry mouth	29.2	26.8	NS
Burning mouth	19.7	16.2	NS

The authors concluded that the hormone had no direct effect upon the oral symptoms. This conclusion is also supported by another study from Canada in 102 patients, 84 of them being women (Grushka[34]). Also in that study, no significant improvement of BMS complaints was obtained after estrogen therapy.

The response of the vaginal epithelium to estrogen, investigated by exfoliative cytology, is quite distinct. In contrast,the response of the oral epithelium is minimal[7]. Local application of estrogen or a combination of estrogen and progesteron on a burning mucosa has been shown to be ineffective[77].

Blood disorders

Iron-deficiency anemia

Iron-deficiency anemia is a rather common symptom. It is the most important causative factor in anemia. It has been estimated that a few percent of all men, and probably 10 to 30% of all women, suffer from iron-deficiency anemia [15].

Iron-deficiency anemia is a sign of a disease, and not a disease itself. Examinations should be undertaken to rule out the possibility of a malignant tumor of the gastrointestinal tract[28]. In women, iron-deficiency anemia can be caused by menstruation.

Iron deficiency can have an insidious onset with gradual progression of fatigue, irritability, palpitations, dizziness, breathlessness, and headache. Other findings suggestive of the presence of iron deficiency include cracks or fissures at the corners of the mouth, a lemon-tinted pallor of the oral mucosa, a smooth, red, painful tongue with atrophy of the papillae, and dysphagia resulting from esophageal stricture or web [28, 44]. The association of dysphagia, angular stomatitis, and lingual papillary abnormalities with iron deficiency anemia is known as the Plummer-Vinson or Paterson-Kelly syndrome.

It has been suggested that iron deficiency plays a role in BMS. In many of the reported cases of a low iron content of the blood, the ferritine level had not been determined, making the diagnosis of iron deficiency questionable [49]. Moreover, it was shown that only 13 of a group of 37 patients with evident iron-deficiency anemia had soreness of the tongue [54].

Pernicious anemia

Pernicious anemia is a megaloblastic anemia caused by a lack of vitamin B_{12}, which is in turn due to a deficiency of the intrinsic factor responsible for the resorption of vitamin B_{12}. The intrinsic factor is a glycoprotein and is secreted by certain parts of the stomach. It has been suggested that pernicious anemia is an autoimmune disorder, because antibodies to the gastric parietal cells are often found in patients with pernicious anemia. The disease has a prevalence of less than 1% and is usually seen after the third decade with equal frequency in both sexes.

Oral symptoms are often present in the form of a burning or itching sensation, a disturbance in taste, intolerance of dentures and, occasionally, dryness of the mouth.

The oral mucosa often will reveal changes consisting of atrophy of the papillae of the dorsum of the tongue. In advanced cases, the dorsum of the tongue has an atrophic, smooth, fiery-red surface[86]. In contrast to the lingual findings in iron deficiency, the tongue in pernicious anemia may show a lobulation.

Vitamin deficiency

In a study in Glasgow of 70 patients suffering from burning mouth, the concentration of a number of vitamins in the blood has been determined (Lamey et al[61]). In 28 patients (40%) a deficiency of vitamins B_1, B_2, B_6, or a combination of these vitamins was shown; no patient was anaemic or iron-deficient. None of the 70 patients showed a deficiency in vitamins A, C, D or E. In a control group consisting of people without BMS, only in 7% was a vitamin deficiency found. The vitamin-deficient group of 28 patients was given appropriate replacement therapy. This consisted of either vitamin B_1 (300 mg per day), vitamin B_2 (20 mg per day in 2 divided doses) or vitamin B_6 (150 mg per day in 3 divided doses). The 6 patients who had combined B-group deficiency received combined therapy. All patients received this therapy for 1 month, at the end of which time repeat vitamin profile assay was undertaken. Patients were asked to grade the overall response at 1 month and 3 months. The nonvitamin-deficient group was given identical vitamin replacement regimes randomly allocated and included 6 patients who received combined treatment. Of the 28 vitamin-deficient patients, 24 were asymptomatic after 1 month and remained so after 3 months. Other BMS patients, without vitamin deficiency, were also given vitamin B therapy. No improvement was reported in any of the patients after 1 month nor after 3 months. The overall results showed that 88% of patients with BMS and proven vitamin deficiency were asymptomatic at 3 months. In contrast, no non-vitamin deficient patient was asymptomatic at 3 months and only approximately 7% were improved.

Hypocalcemia

In a review of BMS several possible causes were mentioned, including serum electrolyte disturbances such as hypocalcemia[109]. No further evidence was provided on this subject and no other reports are available in the literature.

Hypochlorhydria and achlorhydria

Sharp (1976)[89] gave the following description of the oral mucosa in patients with symptoms of BMS: »Characteristic is the red or magenta color of the mucosa. As the condition progresses, the filiform papillae and the submucosa gradually atrophy. Atrophy of the gastric mucosa and submucosa associated with achlorhydria is present in all the patients.« Sharp divided the group into nonachlorhydric and achlorhydric patients. In the nonachlorhydric group, therapy with a special liver fraction tablet was started because of its regenerative effect on mucous membranes. All the nonachlorhydric patients responded through the first year. The achlorhydric patients were given hydrochloric acid supplementation containing 440 mg of betaine hydrochloride, 100 mg of pepsin, and methylcellulose. The average dosage was 1 tablet daily during or after each meal. When symptoms persisted, these patients also were prescribed the liver fraction tablet.

Since Sharp's study was not performed in a so-called double-blind protocol, part of his favorable results should perhaps be ascribed to a placebo effect. No further studies on this subject are available in the literature, except the monograph by Haneke[43] who mentioned that substitution therapy in 12 achlorhydric patients did not reduce the symptoms of BMS. Sharp's conclusion that the hot tongue is a symptom frequently associated with other alimentary tract complaints is not shared by other authors.

Diabetes mellitus

Diabetes mellitus seems to play a role in the etiology of BMS only occasionally, in spite of the report by Brody et al[13]. They described the results of a complete blood count, urinalysis, and an oral 2-hour glucose tolerance test in 142 patients with a variety of oral complaints including 62 patients with a burning sensation. Of all patients studied, 35% had glucose tolerance curves indicative of diabetes. The patients with symptoms of burning had a distribution of glucose tolerance curves similar to the group as a whole. In Brody et al's paper no results of treatment were provided, although it was mentioned that the results in an earlier, somewhat similar study were erratic.

Several authors have reported that symptoms of BMS in diabetic patients in most cases do not decrease after diabetic treatment[18, 75, 32]. In an English study it was shown, more or less by coincidence, that the complaints of BMS patients suffering from diabetes mellitus can be influenced by the type of insulin[7]. In the same report, a low 10% of symptoms of BMS was mentioned in a group of 110 patients being treated for clinical diabetes (see p. 14).

Vascular disturbances

The arterial systems are affected by atherosclerosis in a definite sequence, with involvement of the aorta and carotid arteries preceding that of the coronary, vertebral and intracranial arteries. For a long time little was known about the possible atherosclerotic changes in the lingual artery. In a study of 75 specimens of human cadaver tongues, atheromatous degeneration of the lingual artery branches was found in 69 (92%) of the total 75 cases and in 56 (98%) of the 57 cases over 10 years of age [20]. Atheroma formation was much more prominent in the large and medium-sized branches of the lingual artery than in the smaller segments. There were no statistically significant sex or racial differences with regard to the occurrence of atherosclerosis.

The common finding of atherosclerotic changes of the lingual artery, occurring equally in both sexes, does not provide strong evidence that vascular changes play a role in the etiology of BMS.

Reduced salivary flow rate

It is presumed that, on growing older, the function of the salivary glands decreases, which may cause complaints of dry mouth and which perhaps may predispose to BMS.

In a study of 89 BMS patients the salivary flow rate was measured of »resting saliva« and »stimulated saliva«[101]. A comparison was made with the values of an age- and sex-matched control group of patients without BMS. The secretion of resting saliva was shown to be significantly lower in BMS patients than in the control group. After stimulation a significantly higher secretion in BMS patients was observed, thus reducing the possible role of reduced salivary flow in the etiology of BMS to minor importance.

It seems that a dry mouth can only aggrevate already existing symptoms of burning. Moreover, it should be realized that not all BMS patients suffer from a dry mouth [97].

Side-effects of medication

Older people, being the group that is mainly affected by BMS, often use several medications simultaneously. The reduced physiologic reserve and lower resistance against stress makes this group particularly vulnerable to the noxious effects of these drugs [45].

Zumkley stated that the use of antibiotics in the long term can disturb the intestinal flora, resulting in resorption disturbances, especially of iron and vitamin B_{12}[109].

Several drugs have the capacity to induce dry mouth. A rather extensive list of such xerostomia-inducing drugs is provided by Sreebny and Schwartz[94]. Little is known about the precise mechanism of drug-induced xerostomia. Apparently, the salivary glands can retain their ability to function properly in these circumstances[94].

Discontinuation of diuretics in 5 hypertensive patients with BMS was effective in 3 of them[32].

At any rate, an accurate drug history is essential in the diagnosis of BMS.

Hypothyroidism, immunologic disturbances, rheumatism, erythrocyte sedimentation rate

Apparently, BMS can be due to or associated with hypothyroidism or overtreatment of hyperthyroidism[33].

A number of BMS patients may perhaps suffer from an immunologic disturbance, yet to be further identified[38].

Some authors have noticed that in over 60% of BMS patients the erythrocyte sedimentation rate was slightly raised [34].

At present, none of the above-mentioned findings has led to a better understanding of the etiology or the treatment of BMS.

CHAPTER 6

Neurologic Causes

Pain

In unilateral distribution of pain, attention should be paid not only to a local cause but also to the possibility of a neurologic disturbance. In the latter situation the pain is usually constantly present. In contrast to idiopathic BMS, complaints will increase while speaking, eating and drinking.

Before studying possible neurologic disturbances that can cause BMS, it is necessary to discuss a few aspects of pain. It is beyond the scope of this text to deal with the many aspects of pain in detail. The interested reader is referred to two excellent monographs on this subject [9, 75a].

The definition of pain that is often used is: »An unpleasant sensory and emotional experience associated with actual or potential tissue damage, or described in terms of such damage.« (Intern. Assoc. of Pain, 1986) [53].

Classification of pain

Bell[9] recognizes three main groups of orofacial pain: somatic, neurogenous and psychogenic pain. Furthermore, several clinical pain syndromes are recognized, such as pains of dental origin, pains of muscle origin, temporomandibular joint pains, vascular pains, neurogenous pains, and chronic and psychogenic pains.

Bell discusses BMS under the heading of mucogingival pains of the mouth as an example of superficial somatic pain. Furthermore, the following statement was made: »The location of the pain corresponds to areas of greatest movement, thus revealing the cause as the abrasive effect of the tissues rubbing against themselves and the teeth. Pain location depends on which tissues are being rubbed and where.« In the same paragraph, however, Bell states: »The condition of glossodynia and burning mouth seems to be poorly understood. Much of it is iatrogenic from medication. Anxiety and emotional tension frequently induce or aggravate the condition.«

Bell advocates the use of a topical anesthetic applied to the painful site as a diagnostic test in patients with BMS. Its penetration is too limited to appreciably affect pain sources situated more deeply in the tissues. Heterotopic pains are not affected. Therefore, if application of a topical anesthetic promptly and effectively arrests the pain and induces numbness, the condition truly represents primary hyperalgesia.

Chronic pain

Usually, two types of chronic pain are distinguished:

a. With known nociceptive substrate: nociceptive processes are long existing and psychological and social processes have an inevitable influence on the pain complaints, e.g. chronic pain in patients with a malignancy and chronic pain in other diseases, such as rheuma.

b. Without known nociceptive substrate: nociceptive processes have disappeared in the meantime or are not relevant in relation to the complaint. The pain continues for over six months and psychological and social factors probably play an important role in the maintenance of the complaint. In that case the term »chronic intractable pain« is used. Since the cause of BMS is not well understood, and no nociceptive substrate is known, it is clear that BMS has to be considered a chronic pain without known nociceptive substrate.

Referred pain

Travell and Simons[99] have described the occurrence of a referred pain, caused by spasms of the suprahyoidal muscles, being transmitted via the buccal gingiva of the lower front teeth and then via the incisors and the lingual gingiva. Thereafter, the pain reaches the frontal ventrolateral part of the tongue, which explains the symptoms of BMS. Unfortunately, in the literature only 1 patient has been described who could be treated succesfully by relaxation of the suprahyoidal muscles[58]. In more than 12% of patients suffering from the myofascial pain syndrome, the pain was experienced in the mouth, while the trigger point was located in the medial pterygoid and digastric muscles[27].

Pain threshold

With an electric stimulus the sensitivity threshold of the tongue and palatal mucosa was measured in BMS patients[102]. A comparison was made with the values of control patients without BMS. The sensitivity threshold appeared to be significantly lower in BMS patients than in the control group. Moreover, it was shown that in both groups the sensitivity threshold was higher in people over 70 years of age. It was also remarkable that when BMS patients became asymptomatic, e.g. after dental treatment, the sensitivity threshold had not changed. In an earlier study the pain threshold of the skin was measured in 15 BMS patients and 15 control patients: the cutaneous pain threshold was shown to be the same in both groups[59].

Also in a more recent study the subject of tactile pain and sensory functions in BMS has been dealt with[35, 37].

Psychogenic and social aspects of pain

Laufer described 20 BMS patients in whom local or systemic causes were absent[64]. In his view there is always a psychogenic component involved which influences the pain sensation. In other words: pain and pain sensation are two separate matters. Laufer explicitly points this out to his patients and emphasizes the importance of a good dialogue with the patient. In his experience there is seldom a need for the use of sedatives or analgesics.

The influence of psychogenic and social aspects of pain

sensation are different per patient and per complaint. In practice it is often difficult to distinguish those various aspects.

Neuralgia

Neuralgia of the trigeminal nerve or the glossopharyngeal nerve is a rare phenomenon. It can, however, cause unilateral complaints. Characteristically, the pain is very different from that in BMS and is usually described as sharp, shooting, stabbing, or »like a needle« and commonly lasts from a few seconds to a minute[83]. Among Rushton et al's[83] 217 patients with glossopharyngeal neuralgia, the pain was localized to one or more of the following regions: ear, 155 times; tonsil, 147 times; larynx, 69 times; and tongue 43 times.

The application of a 10% solution of cocaine to the region of the tonsil and pharynx may assist in the correct diagnosis. If the patient finds relief for 1 or 2 hours afterward, the test is considered positive for glossopharyngeal neuralgia.

Postoperative sensory disturbances

A well-known phenomenon is pain in the tongue or a burning or itching sensation after surgical treatment of the tongue or floor of the mouth, during which procedure the lingual nerve has been damaged. Such damage may be unavoidable in some instances,but is always looked upon with suspicion by the patient, being regarded as the result of poor surgical treatment.

CHAPTER 7

Psychogenic Aspects

Introduction

Already in 1920 a possible psychogenic cause of BMS was being mentioned[21]. Also in the more recent literature much attention is paid to possible psychogenic causes. It is interesting to see the various percentages as well as the various criteria that have been used to establish the presence of a nonsomatic cause in the etiology of BMS. For instance, in a study of 57 patients in New York City entitled »Burning mouth«, in 21 of the patients the burning mouth was diagnosed as being psychogenic in origin[107].

Reading superficially, one could conclude that in the aforementioned group of patients about 37% was suffering from a psychogenically-induced disease. On closer study however, 28 patients were included who suffered from a local mucosal disease that was responsible for the oral complaints. Here the nonuniform use of the definition of BMS is misleading since most authors exclude patients with an evident local cause for their symptoms. This means that in the aforementioned study of 57 patients, 28 should have been excluded. Of the remaining 29 patients, 21 were felt to have a psychogenic background to their symptoms, which does not represent 37% but more than 70%.

In Zegarelli's study[107], the diagnosis of a psychogenically-induced disease was established after all other local and systemic disease possibilities had been excluded by a negative clinical picture, negative laboratory findings, and a positive history regarding emotional factors. A few patients had histories of psychiatric illnesses, and others had histories of diseases often related to or associated with stress, namely, peptic ulcer, spastic colon, and hypertension.

It will be clear that, when interpreting the percentages of psychogenic causes of BMS, a critical look should be taken both at the selection of the group of patients and the criteria that have been applied for the establishment of a psychogenic etiologic factor.

Assessment of psychiatric status by questionnaires

Cattell's 16 PF questionnaire (form C)

The Cattell's 16 PF questionnaire (form C) consists of 105 informally worded statements[17]. The questionnaire provides a framework for sampling fundamental behavioral tendencies that have been shown to relate closely to actual behavior.

In a study of 47 patients with BMS, applying Cattell's 16 PF questionnaire, no correlation was found between psychological status and age, sex, initial severity score, cancerophobia, social and domestic circumstances, and denture wearing[60]. Psychological factors were present in more than half of the patients. Anxiety was the most recalcitrant obstacle to cure. Cattell's questionnaires have also been used successfully in other types of dental patients[80, 81].

Clinical interview schedule (CIS)

The clinical interview schedule (CIS) is a semistructured interview designed to be administered by a trained psychiatrist (Goldberg et al)[31].

The CIS makes it possible to determine whether a patient needs psychiatric care and can be categorized according to the International Classification of Disease as proposed by the WHO[72]. The questionnaire seems to provide a reliable measure of psychiatric morbidity among people who do not consider themselves to be mentally ill. The CIS has been applied to patients with facial arthromyalgia and atypical facial pain [24].

One part of the interview consists of an enquiry about any psychiatric symptoms which the patient may have experienced in the preceding week. Goldberg et al used the following nine groups [30]:

Somatic symptoms
Fatigue
Sleep disturbances
Irritability
Lack of concentration
Depression
Anxiety and worry
Obsessions and compulsions
Depersonalization

Eysenck personality questionnaire (EPQ)

The Eysenck personality questionnaire (EPQ) provides a measure to assess extraversion and neuroticism (Eysenck and Eysenck [23]). The EPQ has been used in a study of patients with atypical facial pain [24], and in a study of patients with presumed oral galvanism [55].

General health questionnaire (GHQ)

Zilli et al[108] used the general health questionnaire, 28-item version (GHQ-28) in their screening test for psychiatric illness in patients with oral dysesthesia in whom no organic cause was evident on examination and who had no blood abnormalities in the studies of complete blood count, iron, serum B_{12}, and folate.

The GHQ evaluates the inability to carry out normal functions and has subscales on somatic dysfunction, anxiety and insomnia, social dysfunction, and depression[31]. The scores as measured by Zilli et al using the GHQ-28 show little difference from scores obtained in other pain clinics.

In another study of BMS patients using the 28-item GHQ, 13 patients scored as having psychiatric problems, as compared to 5 in the control group[16]. Most of the patients in whom psychiatric problems were diagnosed had a history of fairly long-standing social and personal difficulties.

Hospital anxiety and depression scale (HAD)

The HAD scale is a self-assessment scale that was designed to detect several disorders of anxiety and depression in nonpsychiatric populations treated at medical clinics[92].

The HAD scale was used in 74 new referrals of BMS, applying a slight modification (Lamey and Lamb[63]). Instead of asking the patients' present feelings, the patients were instructed to report their past week's feelings. Almost 40% had clinically significant anxiety, more than 20% had anxiety scores of borderline significance and almost 40% were not anxious. Following these findings, the authors suggested that the somatic symptoms of burning mouth are at least partly the psychological result of restlessness, tension, and an inherent inability to relax. In the depression subscale, close to 70% of the patients had scores that corresponded to a nondepressive state, while 20% had results of borderline significance. The remaining 10% had both anxiety and depression psychoses. Lamey and Lamb encouraged the use of the HAD scale for objective assessment of the psychological status of patients with BMS. The use of the HAD-scale was also recommended as an ongoing record of the patient's progress at subsequent visits to the clinic.

Irritability depression and anxiety scale (IDA)

In 31 subjects suffering from oral dysesthesia and without detectable organic disease, an IDA scale was used[108]. The IDA is a self-reporting questionnaire that measures depression and anxiety as well as outwardly directed irritability and inwardly directed irritability. The IDA scores were compared with those obtained from the GHQ-28 (see p. 64). The IDA scores obtained in the patients with

65

sore mouth showed a much lower percentage of patients not classified as psychiatric when compared to the GHQ results. The authors concluded that a significant percentage of their subjects were depressed. They added that it is unclear whether the depression is causative or whether it is a result of chronic pain.

Montgomery-Asberg depression rating scale (MADRS)

The Montgomery-Asberg depression rating scale (MADRS) provides a measure of depressive illness (Montgomery and Asberg[74]). It has also been used to measure the changing symptomatology in response to drug treatment[25]. The list of items is shown in Table 10.

TABLE 10. Item list of MADRS (Montgomery and Asberg[74])

1. Apparent sadness
2. Reported sadness
3. Inner tension
4. Reduced sleep
5. Reduced appetite
6. Concentration difficulties
7. Lassitude
8. Inability to feel
9. Pessimistic thoughts
10. Suicidal thoughts

Spielberger state-trait anxiety inventory (STAI-form Y)

The Spielberger state-trait anxiety inventory (form Y) has been used in a group of 154 patients suffering from BMS (Van der Ploeg et al[78]). The state and trait anxiety were clearly above average scores for randomly selected healthy persons, but below the average for psychiatric outpatients.

It was emphasized that the higher scores for anxiety may reflect the psychological consequences of the oral problems rather than the causes.

Psychiatric consultation

Hampf et al[40] reported their experience with psychiatric consultation involving 70 patients with orofacial dysesthesia, which included 18 patients with BMS. Of those 70 patients, 16 cancelled their appointment, 8 of whom belonged to the BMS group. The remaining 54 patients took part in a semistructured psychiatric interview, by a psychiatrist specializing in psychoanalysis who followed DSM III criteria[2] that lasted 1 to 1.5 hour. A control group was recruited and matched for age and sex from patients who were referred for the removal of impacted asymptomatic teeth.The results for BMS are presented in Table 11. In the total group of 54 patients, only 7.4% were mentally healthy, compared with 72.7% of the controls.

TABLE 11. Psychiatric diagnoses of 18 patients with BMS according to the DSM III criteria (Hampf et al[40])

	Number
Paranoid personality disorder	1
Dependent personality disorder	5
Passive-aggressive personality disorder	1
Dysthymic disorder	2
Hypochondriasis	1
Consultation refused	8
Total	18

When signs and symptoms reported by the patient do not correspond with objective findings, Hampf et al recommend referral for consultation either to a multidisciplinary pain clinic or to a psychiatrist, although most patients are not prepared to undergo psychiatric treatment.

Unlike Hampf et al[40], who referred *all* patients for psychiatric consultation, Blasberg et al[11] used selective psychiatric consultation. Based on the history that the patient with orofacial pain gave about his or her complaint four groups were defined on the basis of initial impression by the clinician (Table 12).

TABLE 12. Classification of pain history
(Blasberg et al[11])

Bizarre beliefs
Distorted stories
Persistant themes
Vague and inconsistant histories

Questions to ask patients whose presentation suggests psychiatric illness

When a clinician suspects that psychiatric illness is a factor in the orofacial complaints, Blasberg et al[11] recommend posing the following questions:

»What do you think is causing the pain/discomfort?«

This question often assists in identifying patients with fixed and sometimes delusional beliefs about their symptoms.

»How is your mood?«

This question allows the patient to express his or her mental distress if it is present. If depression is suspected it is important to ask whether suicide has been considered.

As Blasberg et al expect, the chance of suicide is not made more likely by the question, and all too often the reluctance of professionals to ask it increases the risk of missing an opportunity to help these patients before they have to ask for help.

»Have you had any previous medical or dental history of pain (e.g. neck, shoulder, or low back pain), for which medical or surgical treatment was unsuccessful?«

A »yes« to this question may be an indication for psychiatric assessment before irreversible dental treatments are considered in such patients.

»Have you experienced any recent stresses?«

If a major conflict is present at work or in private life, the clinician and the patient may discuss how important this problem is with regard to the current complaint.

Patients' reactions to psychiatric referral

Hampf et al[40] mentioned that, of his 12 psychotic patients, none was aware of being mentally ill. Besides, most patients were not prepared to undergo psychiatric treatment if advised to do so.

Blasberg et al[11] stated that the patient may have a firm belief about his problem that does not include an emotional component. For referral to be successful in this situation, the patient has to accept the possibility that the psychiatric referral may have value for him. Nevertheless, Blasberg et al recognized that some patients simply have fixed beliefs in a somatic cause and reject psychiatric referral.

Facilitating a psychiatric referral

Blasberg et al[11] made a number of suggestions that may be helpful in making a successful (psychiatric) referral, such as:

Inform the patient that this is part of the evaluation and not a termination of the relationship.
If possible, make the appointment for the patient. It provides the patient with a definite commitment that is agreed upon before he leaves the office.

Know the psychiatrist you are recommending. Know what type of evaluation will be performed, so that you may give the patient some indication of what to expect.

Make the mechanics of the referral similar to what you would use to refer the patient to a dental or medical specialist. Indeed, have the mechanics of the referral carried out in a »business as usual« manner.

Oral habits

Quinn reported his experience with 54 patients with BMS, indicating that the cause of burning may be attributed to local irritation and to anxiety resulting in tongue thrusting and tooth clenching[79]. In his series, there were 42 tongue-thrusters, many of whom also were tooth clenchers.

Tesnier, too, explained the complaints of BMS as being the result of apraxic movements of the tongue[98]. Presumably, these movements are related to the »searching« lingual movements of the child in psychological distress.

In the study by Jontell et al[55], oral findings indicating parafunction in a broader sense, i.e. mucosal ridging, petechiae, impressions of the teeth in the tongue, were found in over 50% of patients with oral complaints, including burning sensations, presumed to be caused by galvanism.

Grushka's study of 102 BMS patients provided little or no support for the hypothesis that oral habits are important causative agents in BMS[34].

In the author's experience, oral parafunctions do not seem to be more prevalent among BMS patients than in others, and can hardly be considered a major etiologic factor of the symptoms of burning.

Stereognostic examination

In an attempt to look for reproducible criteria of the BMS, Wagner applied an oral stereognostic test[103]. This test examines the ability of a person to analyze objects in the mouth in a tridimensional way, giving information mainly about sensory ability. In denture-wearing patients the results of such stereognostic examinations are independent of the wearing of dentures.

Patients having their own dentition do better than denture-wearing patients. Patients suffering from BMS needed significantly more time to recognize the objects than persons from a control group, which can perhaps be partly explained by the complaints of burning. Furthermore, BMS patients are often also suffering from xerostomia, which is another factor that may influence the result of the oral stereognostic examination.

No reports are available on this subject in relation to BMS. Apparently, there is no place for stereognostic examination in the routine diagnostic work-up of BMS patients.

Cause and effect relationship

In most studies dealing with psychological aspects in patients suffering from BMS, attempts have been made to objectively assess possible present psychiatric disorders, without claiming a cause and effect relationship in case of the presence of such a disorder.

A few authors firmly defend the thesis that BMS is a symptom of depression and results from psychological stress. Schoenberg stated that the specific psychological stress is a real or threatened loss of a loved person, valued object, or bodily function in individuals who, because of early infantile experience, have a predisposition to depression[84]. As Schoenberg continues: »A dental procedure, viewed unconsciously as an attack on the body, may be a factor in precipitating a depressive reaction with somatic symptoms.«

Haneke stated that almost all his cases of BMS were the result of psychiatric diseases, most often affecting menopausal women with atypical depression[41]. The use of tricyclic antidepressants has been recommended in those circumstances. In Laufer's series of 20 patients a psychological component was »clearly revealed« in each patient[64].

Wagner and Lange[104] reported their experience with 89 patients with BMS and rather categorically denied an important role of psychiatric illness in the etiology of BMS. Van der Ploeg et al[78] demonstrated the presence of a psychological component in BMS patients, but stressed that this finding may not be interpreted as support for a strong psychogenic or psychological factor in the etiology of BMS. The high scores for anxiety and depression may in fact reflect the psychological consequence of the oral problems. A similar statement was made by Zilli et al[108]. Sternbach and Timmermans, too, showed in their group of 113 patients that the neuroticism associated with chronic pain is a result of it, and may be reversible when the pain is reduced or eradicated[95].

Since it has been shown that tricyclic antidepressants may act therapeutically as analgesics[65], a diagnosis of depression as a cause of BMS cannot be concluded from a patient's responsiveness to such medication[36].

Based on personal experience with literally hundreds of patients with BMS who have been referred during the past twenty years to the Department of Oral and Maxillofacial Surgery of the Teaching Hospital of the Free University of Amsterdam, it is tempting to presume the presence of an underlying psychogenic causative factor in a number of patients suffering from BMS. But this does not explain the burning sensation in so many other patients.

The fact of being patient with BMS probably does more to explain the higher scores for anxiety, depression, neuroticism, and neurosomatic lability than the assumption that a certain personality structure is the cause of BMS. To confirm such a relationship one would, among other things, have to perform a prospective study involving a large number of asymptomatic persons of whom the psychiatric status is assessed at entry to the study.

CHAPTER 8

Management

The following guidelines are provided for the »average« patient, above the age of 35-40 years, who seeks medical or dental help for symptoms of bilateral burning or itching of the oral mucosa. BMS-like symptoms in patients under the age of 30 years are extremely uncommon and should be looked upon with caution. This also applies for cases of unilateral, localized symptoms of burning.

History

When a brief history of the nature and duration of the symptoms and an inspection of the oral cavity do not clearly reveal the cause of BMS-like symptoms, a more detailed approach is warranted. When the occasion is not appropriate for either the patient or the doctor, a new appointment should be made, preferably within a week or so.

Although a checklist of questions to ask the patient may be optimum for research purposes, a direct, open communication seems to be preferred by most patients. Of course, there is the risk of forgetting a few items, but this shortcoming can always be taken care of in a further visit.

Symptom history

The symptom history should include a number of items, such as:
1. The nature of the main complaint, as described by the patient.
2. The site distribution of the symptoms, i.e. unilateral versus bilateral, and the specific sites, such as dorsal surface and/or borders of the tongue, tip of the tongue, inner and/or outer surfaces of the upper and lower lip, 73

cheek mucosa, palate etc. In denture-wearing patients, one should ask whether the symptoms are restricted to the denture-bearing mucosa, and whether removal of the dentures affects the symptoms.

3. The course of symptoms, being either constantly present day and night, or arising and worsening during the course of the day. Ask the patient how many days, weeks or months the symptoms have been present and if there have been any remissions.

4. Do the symptoms interfere with eating or drinking; or with falling asleep, or is the patient woken up by his oral problem?

5. The onset of the symptoms as seen from the patient's point of view. Do not ask at this stage about any adverse life experiences.

6. When the patient relates the onset of the symptoms to dental treatment, either of the natural dentition or (partial) dentures, some additional questions may be asked. For instance, how long has the patient been edentulous? Have they had one or more dentures made in the past?

7. Has the patient consulted any other doctor in the past about his symptoms? What examinations or laboratory studies have been performed and what treatment has been instituted, or what advice given?

8. Many patients do not dare to inform the clinician as to possible consultations that they have sought outside the regular medical or dental care services, being afraid to be humiliated. Help the patient to overcome this reluctance.

9. The presence of other oral problems, such as a dry mouth and an altered taste or even a lack of taste.

10. The presence of other somatic complaints, such as gastrointestinal symptoms, headaches, migraine, neck and/or backache, etc.

11. Which activities, events or measures ease or aggravate the problem?

12. How do relatives and close friends react to the patient's complaints?

Medical history

The medical history is another important part of the history-taking and should include items such as:

1. Possible other present illnesses or illnesses experienced in the past, including surgery and other treatment modalities. Touch upon any psychiatric treatment only when this subject is brought up spontaneously by the patient himself.
2. Is the patient aware of any allergy to food substances or did he ever experience some other allergic reactions?

Drug history

Especially in patients who also complain of xerostomia, the taking of an accurate drug history is mandatory, including questions such as:

1. What medication is the patient taking (present and in the past) and for what indication?
2. Questions about the possible use of sleeping pills, tranquillizers, etc. should be raised tactfully, avoiding giving the patient the impression of being categorized as 'a psychiatric case'.

Oral examination

In all circumstances, irrespective of the nature and exact distribution of the symptoms, a thorough inspection of the entire oral cavity, including the tongue, should be carried out under the appropriate conditions, as has been described on p. 22.

A localized burning or itching sensation can be the first sign of a malignant or premalignant mucosal lesion. Ignoring the importance of such symptoms or overlooking subtle but ominous mucosal changes may have dramatic sequelae. Besides, there is a large number of benign lesions and conditions of the oral mucosa that may produce

BMS-like symptoms. These lesions have been briefly discussed in Chapter 4.

It is striking that, in most patients whose complaints include xerostomia, a normal or sometimes even a superfluity of saliva is found at inspection. However, one should refrain from making statements such as: »How can you complain of a dry mouth? There is plenty of saliva.«

The result of the oral examination is more or less decisive for the future management of the patient. The two further pathways in the management of the symptoms are based on the presence or absence of clinically visible changes of the oral mucosa (Table 13).

Positive oral findings

In case of clinically visible changes in the oral mucosa one has to verify whether the nature and anatomic distribution of the complaints correspond with the mucosal changes. If not, such mucosal changes, e.g. geographic tongue, may be of little or no importance with regard to the BMS-like symptoms.

When the site of the complaints does correspond with the clinical visible mucosal changes, several possibilities arise. One may be dealing with a primary lesion or condition of the oral mucosa, which in many cases requires the taking of a biopsy. Furthermore, the possibility of an allergic reaction to a restorative dental material is to be ruled out, preferably by cutaneous patch testing (see p. 47). Tests for galvanism may be considered as well (see p. 46).

When the mucosal changes are limited to the denture-bearing tissues, attention should be focused upon the various aspects of the dentures, such as stability, occlusal height, denture hygiene (Candida albicans), and possible allergy to one or more compounds used in denture base material, as is discussed on p. 43.

Finally, in the presence of clinically visible changes in the color or the texture of the oral mucosa, the possibility of an underlying systemic disease should be considered, such as iron deficiency (see p. 52) or pernicious anemia

TABLE 13. Decision tree in the management of patients

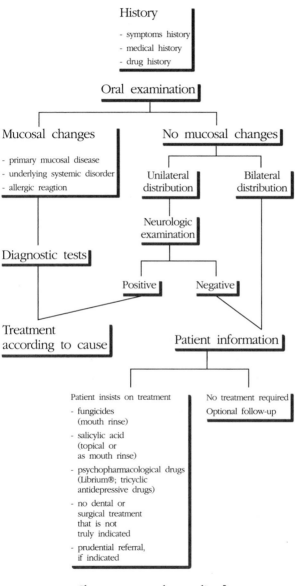

History
- symptoms history
- medical history
- drug history

Oral examination

Mucosal changes
- primary mucosal disease
- underlying systemic disorder
- allergic reagtion

No mucosal changes

Unilateral distribution

Bilateral distribution

Neurologic examination

Diagnostic tests

Positive

Negative

Treatment according to cause

Patient information

Patient insists on treatment
- fungicides (mouth rinse)
- salicylic acid (topical or as mouth rinse)
- psychopharmacological drugs (Librium®; tricyclic antidepressive drugs)
- no dental or surgical treatment that is not truly indicated
- prudential referral, if indicated

No treatment required
Optional follow-up

Show your understanding

(see p. 52). Blood examination in these circumstances will include:

complete blood count (CBC)
mean corpuscular volume (MCV)
mean corpuscular hemoglobin (MCH)
white cell count
vitamin B_{12} (one may consider including B_1, B_2, and
  B_6 as well; see p. 53)
folate (serum and red blood cells)
serum iron
total iron binding capacity (TIBC)
ferritin levels and % transferrin saturation

Treatment should be instituted according to the established diagnosis.

Negative oral findings

When no oral mucosal lesions can be detected during inspection (Fig. 16), a large number of items and questions need to be focused upon:

1. Cytologic or histologic examination of the mucosa at the site of burning or any other oral site does not contribute in any way to the further management of the patient. The same applies to the taking of oral smears for culture purposes (e.g. Candida albicans).

2. In patients having their own dentition the question may arise as to whether galvanism is present. Mainly based on findings from the literature (see p. 46) galvanism is unlikely to play a major role in the etiology of BMS, especially in the absence of visible mucosal changes. Therefore, routine measuring of the currents at various sites in the dentition is not warranted. A more or less similar view is held with regard to malocclusion (see p. 47) and oral hygiene (see p. 47).

3. In the absence of mucosal changes referral for allergic studies is not indicated (see p. 47)

4. In patients wearing partial or complete dentures, atten-

tion should be paid to proper occlusion, articulation, stability, etc. (see p. 42). In the absence of clinically visible mucosal changes examination for possible sensitivity to acryl resin is not indicated (see p. 43).

5. Measuring of the salivary flow rate and the electrolyte values of the saliva does not essentially contribute to the management of the symptoms of BMS and, therefore, should not be performed routinely (see p. 56).

6. Routine blood examination, plasma glucose and urinalysis for glucose should not be performed routinely, but only when requested by the patient. The same policy can be followed with regard to the determination of estrogen levels in women, and with regard to other factors such as rheumatoid factor (RF) and antinuclear factor (AF). Based on a rather recent paper in the literature, the vitamin B status, i.e. B_1, B_2 and B_6, may be worth investigating (see p. 53). Supplementation therapy is only indicated in deficient patients.

7. In the absence of an organic causative factor the possibility of side-effects of medication, if any, should be considered (see p. 56). Drug substitution can, indeed, be considered as part of the diagnostic workup. The object of drug substitution is to identify alterative drugs which preserve the primarily desired effect of the prescribed medicament, but which are less able to induce oral side-effects such as dry mouth[94]. When no alternative medication is available a lowered dosis may be helpful. Furthermore, several smaller, more frequently taken doses may alleviate the adverse effects. Preferably, drugs already being prescribed by another colleague should not be changed without prior consultation with that colleague, irrespective of the type of drug.

Management of idiopathic BMS

At this stage the patient needs detailed information about his problem. If possible, the spouse or any other close relative should be present during the further dialogue with 79 the patient. The information should at least contain the basic elements of the syndrome.

Patient information

1. BMS is a rather uncommon, but definitely not exceptional syndrome, that affects menopausal and post-menopausal women much more often than men. Not many doctors and dentists are familiar with the signs and symptoms of the syndrome, which may account for the various and often diverse advice that already may have been given to the patient in the past.

2. In many cases the etiology is unknown, which may result in a wide range of beliefs held by the patient, including the fear of an underlying malignant disease. By explicitly mentioning the unlikelihood of the latter, a number of patients will be completely reassured and will not require any further treatment or follow-up: »Now I know that it is a benign condition I think I can live with it.«

3. Another often-held belief by the patient is a possible allergy for food, toothpaste, chewing gum etc, which, as has been mentioned, is rarely if ever the cause of BMS complaints. The same holds true for smoking habits and the use of alcohol.

4. As in other complaints or diseases for which no distinct cause can be found, the possibility of an underlying psychogenic cause is sometimes brought up. The view should be expressed that it is far more likely that long lasting and intensive symptoms may affect someone's psychological status rather than the reverse. Depending on the patient's reaction to this statement one may elaborate on the subject of nonsomatic causes of diseases in general and of BMS in particular. Some patients themselves wonder whether stress or emotional disturbances may be of importance in relation to their complaints. Again, one may inform the patient that stress or nervousness may aggravate the symptoms, but

that it is difficult to conceive that nervousness plays a major role in the symptoms arising.

5. Even when patients openly admit that they have gone through, or are still involved in, serious and adverse life events, caution is warranted in further exploring these subjects. When the clinician is not properly trained to perform a professional psychological counseling, the patient may finally feel more or less cheated after having revealed his personal problems and emotions. Rather, one may recommend the patient to think it over and to consider the possibility of a psychiatric consultation. Chances further remain that a patient will experience such consultation as extremely beneficial in many respects other than his complaints of burning.

6. In conjunction with the previous item the possible role of oral habits, such as tongue-thrusting or tooth-clenching should be considered (see p. 70). Tesnier even advised addressing therapy in all cases of idiopathic BMS first of all to the distress, followed by immobilization excercises of the tongue, giving rise to consciousness of movements that up to then were unconscious[98]. Tesnier advocates keeping the tip of the tongue against the lingual or palatal surfaces of the incisors for 30 seconds, for 1 minute, for 2 minutes etc, until the patient really masters the movements of his tongue.

7. It should be made clear to the patient that, in view of the poorly understood etiology of BMS, treatment can only be sypmtomatic at the best.

8. Even in patients who suffer from BMS for many months or even years, the symptoms may disappear spontaneously at varying times. On the other hand, the symptoms may persist more or less lifelong in quite a number of patients. However, it is the author's experience that in the majority of such cases the patients have become somewhat used to the symptoms and have given up seeking treatment. In fact, there are no well-documented long-term follow-up studies of large numbers of patients suffering from idiopathic BMS[62].

No active treatment required by the patient

After being properly informed about the various aspects of BMS, some patients do not further insist on any type of treatment. Especially those who were afraid they were suffering from an underlying malignant disease may feel extremely relieved. In any case, patients should be offered a follow-up visit after 3-6 months. Some will happily accept, while others will question the use of such a visit in view of the expected chronicity of the syndrome.

Active treatment required by the patient

In spite of being informed about the lack of therapeutic measures, a number of patients will insist on further treatment or diagnostic tests. With regard to the latter, it seems acceptable to entertain the patient's request to some extent, e.g. for allergic tests or oral smears for culturing, even if the clinician does not feel the need for such tests. Such tests may be costly, but will not harm the patient in any way.

The clinician should be reluctant to follow a patient's wish for any dental or surgical procedure of questionable indication. One rather refuses treatment under such circumstances, accepting the patient's disapproval as to the clinician's lack of competence than being accused by the patient afterwards of having performed a treatment that has worsened his complaints. (»Doctor, when I came to your office I had a bad oral problem, but I could stand it. Now you have treated me, my problem has become very much worse. What have you done?«). The patient-doctor relationship often becomes disrupted in such circumstances. The common orally-administered analgesics may relieve the symptoms for some hours. However, most patients with BMS do not want to use such analgesics, disliking the idea of having to take quite a number of pills every day for a more or less indefinite period of time.

Some patients, even when they understand that there is no uniform treatment available, will insist on a prescription for a mouthrinse or will ask for some type of drug therapy. For this purpose one may consider prescribing, for some weeks or even a few months, fungicides, such as Nystatin®, even when no culture is performed or in case of a negative result of such culture (see p. 23).

Another, somewhat empirical prescription may consist of local application at the burning sites for about 10 seconds of a solution of 7% salicylic acid in 70% alcohol, soaked in cotton pellets, as has been used for palliative treatment of geographic tongue (Henricsson and Axell[47]). Immediately afterwards, patients should rinse their mouths with water. This procedure can be carried out several times a day. Instead of local application of the salicylic acid solution, a mouth rinse can be prepared, again empirically and not based on the results of a double-blind controlled study. Even when its effect is based on a placebo, it is gratifying to be able to prescribe a mouthrinse that a patient did not have before (Table 14).

TABLE 14. Mouth rinse for symptoms of BMS

R.

Salicylic acid	300 mg
Vanilline	10 mg
Alcohol 96% in water	5 ml
Solutio sorbitol	20 ml
Purified water, q.s. ad	100 ml

Make solution
  Sig: Use 1 dessertspoonful undiluted as a
       mouthwash twice a day for 1 minute,
       after meals.
       Do not swallow.

The use of a viscous solution of lidocaine hydrochloride 2% in a carboxymethylcellulose sodium and water vehicle with color and flavor is not very much appreciated by BMS patients. Apparently, the analgesic effect is of very short duration.

In patients who do not benefit from any of the suggested treatment modalities discussed so far, the possibility of the prescription of psychopharmacologic drugs may be considered. It largely depends on the qualifications of the clinician as to whether he is the appropriate person to prescribe drugs such as Librium® [35] or one of the tricyclic antidepressive drugs.

A number of patients will reject the proposition of drug therapy, and prefer to manage their problem without such therapy.

When the clinician or the patient feels the need for referral to another specialist, help the patient to avoid getting lost in a doctor's circuit, being transferred from one to the other.

Do not raise the patient's expectations of a consultation with another doctor too highly. This may only aggravate the disappointment when no solution to the problem can be offered by the other doctor.

In any case, offer the patient the possibility of continuing the communication with you about his problem. This can be done by making a firm appointment for a follow-up visit in the immediate future or by suggesting that the patient can call for an appointment whenever he feels the need for it.

Show your understanding and commitment to the patient's problem. An apparently insoluble problem will then become a manageable one in the majority of cases.

References

The collection of references ended 1 January 1990.

1. Ali A, Bates JF, Reynolds AJ, et al. The burning mouth sensation related to the wearing of acrylic dentures: an investigation. Br Dent J 1986; 161: 444-7.
2. American Psychiatric Association (APA). Diagnostic and statistical manual of mental disorders, 3rd edn. Washington DC, 1983.
3. Axéll T. A prevalence study of oral mucosal lesions in an adult Swedish population. Thesis. Odontol Revy 1976; 27: Suppl. 36.
4. Axéll T, Holmstrup P, Kramer IRH, et al. International seminar on oral leukoplakia and associated lesions related to tobacco habits. Community Dent Oral Epidemiol 1984; 12: 146-54.
5. Axéll T, Nilner K, Nilsson, B. Clinical evaluation of patients referred with symptoms related to oral galvanism. Swed Dent J 1983; 7: 169-78.
6. Bàno'czy J, Szabó L, Csiba A. Migratory glossitis: a clinical-histological review of seventy cases. Oral Surg, Oral Med, Oral Pathol 1975; 39: 113-21.
7. Basker RM, Sturdee DW, Davenport JC. Patients with burning mouths. A clinical investigation of causative factors, including the climacteric and diabetes. Br Dent J 1978; 145: 9-16.
8. Bäurle G, Schönberger A. Glossodynie-Indikation zur Epikutantestung? Z Hautkr 1986; 61: 1175-84.
9. Bell WE. Orofacial Pains. Classification, Diagnosis, Management. 4th edn. Chicago-London-Boca Raton: Year Book Medical Publ Inc., 1989.
10. Bergman M, Ginstrup O, Nilsson B. Potentials of and currents between dental metallic restorations. Scand J Dent Res 1982; 90: 404-8.
11. Blasberg B, Remick RA, Miles JE. The psychiatric referral in dentistry: indications and mechanisms. Oral Surg, Oral Med, Oral Pathol 1983; 56: 368-71.
12. Breustedt von A, Höcker M. Zungenveränderungen beim alten Menschen. Zahn-, Mund- und Kieferheilkunde 1978; 66: 589-97.
13. Brody HA, Prendergast JJ, Silverman S. The relationship between oral symptoms, insulin release, and glucose intolerance. Oral Surg, Oral Med, Oral Pathol 1971; 31: 777-82.
14. Brooke RI. Atypical odontalgia. Oral Surg, Oral Med, Oral Pathol 1980; 49: 196-9.
15. Brown EB. Iron deficiency anemia. In: Wynn-Gaarden JB, Smith LH, (eds). Cecil's textbook of medicine. 16th edn. Philadelphia: WB Saunders Company, 1982: 844-851

16. Browning S, Hislop S, Scully C, et al. The association between burning mouth syndrome and psychological disorders. Oral Surg, Oral Med, Oral Pathol 1987; 64: 171-4.

17. Cattell RB, Eber HW, Tatsuoka M. Handbook for the 16 PF Questionnaire. Champaign, Illinois: Institute of Personality and Ability Testing, 1970.

18. Chinn H, Brody H, Silverman S, et al. Glucose tolerance in patients with oral symptoms. J Oral Ther Pharmacol 1966; 2: 261-9.

19. Chosak A, Zadik D, Eidelman E. The prevalence of scrotal tongue and geographic tongue in 70 359 Israeli schoolchildren. Community Dent Oral Epidemiol 1974; 2: 253-7.

20. Dreizen S, Levy BM, Stern MH, et al. Human lingual atherosclerosis. Arch Oral Biol 1976; 19: 813-6.

21. Engman MF. Burning tongue. Arch Dermatol Syphil 1920; 6: 137-8.

22. Epstein JB, Pearsall NN, Truelove EL. Oral candidiasis: effects of antifungal therapy upon clinical signs and symptoms, salivary antibody, and mucosal adherence of Candida albicans. Oral Surg, Oral Med, Oral Pathol 1981; 51: 32-6.

23. Eysenck HJ, Eysenck SBG. Manual of the Eysenck Personality Questionnaire. London: Hodder and Stoughton, 1975.

24. Feinmann C, Harris M. Psychogenic facial pain. Part 1. The clinical presentation. Br Dent J 1984; 156: 165-8.

25. Feinmann C, Harris M. Psychogenic facial pain. Part 2. Management and prognosis. Br Dent J 1984; 156: 205-8.

26. Ferguson MM, Carter J, Boyle P, et al. Oral complaints related to climacteric symptoms in oophorectomized women. J R Soc Med 1981; 74: 491-8.

27. Friction JR, Kroening R, Haley D, et al. Myofascial pain syndrome of the head and neck: a review of clinical characteristics of 164 patients. Oral Surg, Oral Med, Oral Pathol 1985; 60: 615-23.

28. Gallagher FJ, Baxter DL, Denobile J, et al. Glossodynia, iron deficiency anemia, and gastrointestinal malignancy. Report of a case. Oral Surg, Oral Med, Oral Pathol 1988; 65: 130-3.

29. Glick D, Ben-Aryeh H, Gutman D, et al. Relation between idiopathic glossodynia and salivary flow rate and content. Int J Oral Maxillofac Surg 1976; 5: 161-5.

30. Goldberg DP, Cooper B, Eastwood MR, et al. A standard psychiatric interview for use in community surveys. Br J Prev Soc Med 1970; 24: 18-22.

31. Goldberg DP, Hillier VF. A scaled version of the General Health Questionnaire. Psychol Med 1978; 8: 1-7.

32. Gorsky M, Silverman S, Chinn H. Burning mouth syndrome: a review of 98 cases. J Oral Med 1987; 42: 7-9.

33. Goss AN. Sore tongue. New Zeal Dent J 1973; 69: 194-201.

34. Grushka M. Clinical features of burning mouth syndrome. Oral Surg, Oral Med, Oral Pathol 1987; 63: 30-6.

35. Grushka M, Sessle BJ. Demographic data and pain profile of burning mouth syndrome (BMS). J Dent Res 1985; 64: 1648.

36. Grushka M, Sessle BJ. Burning mouth syndrome: A historical review. Clin J Pain 1987; 2: 245-52.

37. Grushka M, Sessle BJ, Howley TP. Psychophysical assessment of tactile pain and thermal sensory functions in burning mouth syndrome. Pain 1987; 28: 169-84.

38. Grushka M, Shupak R, Sessle BJ. A rheumatological investigation of 27 patients with Burning Mouth Syndrome. J Dent Res 1986; 26: 533.

39. Hampf G. Dilemma in treatment of patients suffering from orofacial dysaesthesia. Int J Oral Maxillofac Surg 1987; 16: 397-401.

40. Hampf G, Vikkula J, Ylipaevalniemi P, et al. Psychiatric disorders in orofacial dysaesthesia. Int J Oral Maxillofac Surg 1987; 16: 402-7.

41. Haneke E. Psychische Aspekte der Glossodynie. Dtsch med Wschr 1978; 103: 1302-5.

42. Haneke E. Das Krankheitsbild der sogenannten Glossodynie. Eine Synopsis klinischer und histomorphologischer Untersuchungen unter besonderer Berücksichtigung vergleichenden histologischen und fluoreszens-histochemischen Befunde. Med Habil Schrift, Erlangen, 1978

43. Haneke E. Zungen- und Mundschleimhautbrennen; Klinik, Differentialdiagnose, Aetiologie, Therapie. Munchen-Wien: Carl Hanser Verlag 1980.

44. Harris M, Davies G. Psychiatric disorders. In: Jones JH, Mason DK (eds). Oral manifestations of systemic disease. London: WB Saunders, 1980: 439-53.

45. Hazzard WR. Leading the health care team for the elderly. In: Petersdorf RG, et al. (eds). Harrison's Principles of Internal Medicine. New York: McGraw-Hill Book Co., 1983.

46. Helfman RJ. The treatment of geographic tongue with topical retin-A-solution. Cutis 1979; 24: 179-80.

47. Henricsson V, Axéll T. Palliative treatment of geographic tongue. Swed Dent J 1980; 4: 129-34.

48. Hollander L. Galvanic burns of the oral mucosa. JAMA 1932; 99: 393-4.

49. Hughes-Jones NC. Lecture notes in haematology. 3rd edn. Oxford: Blackwell Scientific Publications, 1979.

50. Hughes AM, Hunter S, Still D, et al. Psychiatric disorders in a dental clinic. Br Dent J 1989; 166: 16-9.

51. Hugoson A. Results obtained from patients referred for the investigation of complaints related to oral galvanism. Swed Dent J 1986; 10: 15-28.

52. Hume WJ. Geographic stomatitis: a critical review. J Dent 1975; 3: 24-43.

53. International Association for the Study of Pain, Subcommittee on Taxonomy. Classification of chronic pain: descriptions of chronic pain syndromes and definitions of pain terms. Pain 1986 (suppl. 3).

54. Jacobs A, Cavill I. The oral lesions of iron deficiency anaemia: pyridoxine and riboflavin status. Br J Haematol 1968; 14: 291-4.

55. Jontell M, Haraldson T, Persson L-O, et al. An oral and psychosocial examination of patients with presumed oral galvanism. Swed Dent J 1985; 9: 175-85.

56. Kaaber S, Thulin H, Nielsen E. Skin sensitivity to denture base materials in the burning mouth syndrome. Contact Dermatitis 1979; 5: 90-6.

87

57. Katz J, Benoliel R, Leviner E. Burning mouth sensation associated with fusospirochetal infection in edentulous patients. Oral Surg, Oral Med, Oral Pathol 1986; 62: 152-4.

58. Konzelman JL. Glossodynia: a case report. J Craniomand Pract 1985; 3: 82-3.

59. Kutscher AH, Chilton NW. Dolorimetric evaluation of idiopathic glossodynia. New York State Dent J 1952; 18: 31-4.

60. Lamb AB, Lamey P-J, Reeve PE. Burning mouth syndrome: psychological aspects. Br Dent J 1988; 165: 256-60.

61. Lamey P-J, Hammond A, Allam BF, et al. Vitamin status of patients with burning mouth syndrome and the response to replacement therapy. Br Dent J 1986; 160: 81-4.

62. Lamey P-J, Lamb AB. Aetiological factors in burning mouth syndrome: A prospective study. Br Med J 1988; 296: 1243-6.

63. Lamey P-J, Lamb AB. The usefulness of the HAD scale in assessing anxiety and depression in patients with burning mouth syndrome. Oral Surg, Oral Med, Oral Pathol 1989; 67: 390-2.

63a Lamey PJ, Lewis MAO. Oral medicine in practice: burning mouth syndrome. Br Dent J 1989; 167: 197-200.

64. Laufer Ch. Aspects psychosomatique des glossodynies. Actual Odontostomatol 1974; 108: 661-6.

65. Lee R, Spencer PSJ. Antidepressants and pain: a review of the pharmacological data supporting the use of certain tricyclins in chronic pain. J Int Med Res 1977; 5: Suppl 146-56.

66. van Loon LAJ, Elsas PW, van Joost Th, et al. Test battery for metal allergy in dentistry. Contact Dermatitis 1986; 14: 158-61.

67. Luhn J-P, Donath K, Haneke E. Veränderungen der Lippenspeicheldrüsen bei Glossodynie. HNO 1981; 29: 10-6.

68. Lundström IMC. Incidence of diabetes mellitus in patients with oral lichen planus. Int J Oral Maxillofac Surg 1983; 12: 147-52.

69. Lundström IMC. Allergy and corrosion of dental materials in patients with oral lichen planus. Int J Oral Maxillofac Surg 1984; 13: 16-24.

70. Main DMG, Basker RM. Patients complaining of a burning mouth. Further experience in clinical assessment and management. Br Dent J 1983; 154: 206-11.

71. McCabe JF, Basker RM. Tissue sensitivity to acrylic resin. A method of measuring the residual monomer content and its clinical application. Br Dent J 1976; 140: 347-50.

72. Mental Disorders: Glossary and Guide to their Classification in accordance with the ninth revision of the International Classification of Diseases. Geneva: WHO 1978.

73. Mock D, Frydman W, Gordon AS. Atypical facial pain: A retrospective study. Oral Surg, Oral Med, Oral Pathol 1985; 59: 472-4.

74. Montgomery SA, Asberg M. A new depression scale designed to be sensitive to change. Br J Psychiatry 1979; 134: 382-9.

75. Oles RD. Prediabetic glossodynia responsive to diet. J Michig Dent Ass 1979; 61: 305-7.

75a Petersen JK, Milgrom P. Pain relief in the orofacial regions. Copenhagen: Munksgaard, 1989.

88

76. Pindborg JJ. Atlas of Diseases of the Oral Mucosa. 4th edn. Copenhagen: Munksgaard, 1985: 234.

77. Pisanti S, Rafaely B, Polishuk WZ. The effect of steroid hormones on buccal mucosa of menopausal women. Oral Surg, Oral Med, Oral Pathol 1975; 40: 346-53.

78. van der Ploeg HM, van der Wal N, Eijkman MAJ, et al. Psychological aspects of patients with burning mouth syndrome. Oral Surg, Oral Med, Oral Pathol 1987; 63: 664-8.

79. Quinn JH. Glossodynia. J Am Dent Ass 1965; 70: 1418-21.

80. Reeve P, Stafford GD, Hopkins R. The use of Cattell's personality profile in patients who have had preprosthetic surgery. J Dent 1982; 10: 121-30.

81. Reeve P, Watson C, Stafford GD. The role of personality in the management of complete denture patients. Br Dent J 1984; 156: 356-62.

82. Remick RA, Blasberg B, Barton JS et al. Ineffective dental and surgical treatment associated with atypical facial pain. Oral Surg, Oral Med, Oral Pathol 1983; 55: 355-8.

83. Rushton JG, Stevens JC, Miller RH. Glossopharyngeal (Vago-glossopharyngeal) Neuralgia. Arch Neural 1981; 38: 201-5.

83a Samaranayaka LP, Lamb AB, Lamey P-J, MacFarlane TW. Oral carriage of *Candida* species and coliforms in patients with burning mouth syndrome. J Oral Pathol Med 1989; 18: 233-5.

84. Schoenberg B. Psychogenic aspects of the burning mouth.New York State Dent J 1967; 33: 467-73.

85. Scott J, Huskisson EL. Graphic representation of pain. Pain 1976; 2: 175-84.

86. Schmitt RJ, Sheridan PJ, Rogers RS. Pernicious anemia with associated glossodynia. JADA 1988; 117: 838-40.

87. Schroff J. Painful (burning) tongue of foliate papilla (lymphoid follicle). J Oral Maxillofac Surg 1960; 18: 207-17.

88. Sharp GE. The hot tongue syndrome. Etiology and treatment. Arch. Otolaryngol 1967; 85: 112-4.

89. Sharp GS. Burning tongue in menopause - An indicator of alimentary tract dysfunction. JAMA 1976; 235: 307.

90. Sindet-Pedersen S, Petersen JK, Götzsche PC. Incidence of pain conditions in dental practice in a Danish county. Community Dent Oral Epidemiol 1985; 13: 244-6.

91. Sluder G. Some clinical observations on the lingual tonsil concerning goitre, glossodynia and facial infection. Am J Med Sci 1918; 156: 248-52.

92. Snaith RP, Taylor CM. Rating scales for depression and anxiety: A current perspective. Br J Clin Pharmac 1985; 19: 175-205.

93. Spens E. Untersuchungen zum Ursachenkomplex des Mundschleimhaut- und Zungenbrennen. Stomatol (DDR) 1981; 31: 329-39.

94. Sreebny LM, Schwartz SS. A reference guide to drugs and dry mouth. Gerodontology 1986; 5: 75-99.

95. Sternbach RA, Timmermans G. Personality changes associated with reduction of pain. Pain 1975; 1: 177-81.

89

96. Svedja J, Janota M. Scanning electron microscopy of the papillae folia-tae of the human tongue. Oral Surg, Oral Med, Oral Pathol 1974; 37: 208-16.

97. Syrjänen S, Piironen P, Yli-Urpo A. Salivary content of patients with subjective symptoms resembling galvanic pain. Oral Surg, Oral Med, Oral Pathol 1984; 58: 387-93.

98. Tesnier D. Quelques idées sur l'étiologie et le traitement des glosso-dynies. Revue de Stomatol 1975; 76: 417-21.

99. Travell JG, Simons DG. Myofascial Pain and Dysfunction: The Trigger Point Manual. Baltimore: Williams and Wilkins, 1983: 273-81.

100. Wagner I-V. Ein Beitrag zur Deutung und Differenzierung der Be-griffe Stomatitis prothetica und Glossalgie bzw. Stomatodynie. Sto-matol (DDR) 1979; 29: 679-83.

101. Wagner I-V. Möglichkeiten der Objektivierung des Syndroms der Glossalgie und Stomatodynie. 1. Mitteilung: Quantitative Speichel-messungen. Zahn-, Mund- u. Kieferheilkd 1984; 72: 211-6.

102. Wagner I-V. Möglichkeiten der Objektivierung des Syndroms der Glossalgie und Stomatodynie. 2. Mitteilung: Untersuchungen zur Sensibilitätsschwelle. Zahn-, Mund- u Kieferheilkd 1984; 72: 316-9.

103. Wagner I-V. Möglichkeiten der Objektivierung des Syndroms der Glossalgie und Stomatodynie. 3. Mitteilung: Stereognostische Unter-suchungen. Zahn-, Mund- u Kieferheilkd 1984; 72: 425-30.

104. Wagner I-V, Lange E. Zur Frage der psychischen Disposition bei Glossalgie- und Stomatodynie-Patienten. ZWR 1984; 93: 216-8.

105. Wakkers-Garritsen BG, Timmer LH, Nater JP. Etiological factors in the denture sore mouth syndrome: an investigation of 24 patients. Contact Dermatitis 1975; 1: 337-43.

106. Willemsen WL, Opdam NJM, Verdonschot EHAM. Tandheelkunde-onderwijs met betrekking tot pijn: een probleemverkenning. Ned Tijdschr Tandheelkd 1987; 94: 444-7.

107. Zegarelli DJ. Burning mouth: an analysis of 57 patients. Oral Surg, Oral Med, Oral Pathol 1984; 58: 34-8.

108. Zilli C, Brooke RI, Lau CL, et al. Screening for psychiatric illness in patients with oral dysesthesia by means of the General Health Ques-tionnaire - twenty eight item version (GHQ-28) and the Irritability, Depression and Anxiety Scale (IDA). Oral Surg, Oral Med, Oral Pathol 1989; 67: 384-9.

109. Zumkley H. Prothesenunverträglichkeit aus internistischer Sicht. Dtsch zahnärtzl Z 1976; 31: 8-9.

Subject index